I0455918

The All Home Care Matters Official Family Caregivers' Guide

by

Lance A. Slatton

Copyright 2024. Lance A. Slatton . All rights reserved.

ISBN-13: (hardcover)
ISBN-13: (paperback)
ISBN-13: (ebook)
ISBN-13: (audiobook)

No part of this book may be reproduced in any form or by any electronic or mechanical means including information storage and retrieval systems, without permission in writing from the author. The only exception is by a reviewer, who may quote short excerpts in a review.

Although the author and publisher have made every effort to ensure that the information in this book was correct at press time, the author and publisher do not assume and hereby disclaim any liability to any party for any loss, damage, or disruption caused by errors or omissions, whether such errors or omissions result from negligence, accident, or any other cause.

This publication is designed to provide accurate and authoritative information with regard to the subject matter covered. It is sold with the understanding that the publisher is not engaged in rendering professional services. If legal advice or other expert assistance is required, the services of a competent professional should be sought.

The fact that an organization or website is referred to in this work as a citation and/or a potential source of further information does not mean that the author or the publisher endorses the information the organization or website may provide or recommendations it may make.

Please remember that Internet websites listed in this work may have changed or disappeared between when this work was written and when it is read.

The dedication of this book is to:

To my mom who without you I would not be who I am today. I love you more than words could describe.

To my grandparents and role-models "Pops & Ooh-Ooh" who always lead by example and will always be close to my heart.

To my beautiful wife that is always there for me and our family.

Finally, to the greatest joys in my life –"Roo, Goose, and Mad Dog"

The love for each of you is indescribable and immeasurable.

I am lucky to have been given the opportunity to be your dad. The joy and pride I have watching each of you grow is the greatest gift that you could ever give to me.

Man Behind the Book

The All Home Care Matters Official Family Caregivers' Guide is not your ordinary book thanks to the author Lance A. Slatton. You see, as the saying goes "the woman behind the man," well Lance is "the man behind the book!"

Knowing Lance as I do, his skin is probably crawling right now as he reads this, but I feel it's important for people to know the integrity of the author.

Lance is the definition of humble, and hates getting attention; yet due to his personality, skillsets, competitive nature, and character, he draws attention. He is a true servant of people and is inclusive, and respectful, and freely gives his time and insights to lift others.

If you asked Lance what he does he would probably say he is a senior case manager at Enriched Life Home Care Services and that he hosts the All Home Care Matters podcast & YouTube show and that he Co-Hosts The Caregivers' Journal with Denise Brown and also

Co-hosts Conscious Caregiving with L & L with me. This is all true, but not the whole story.

You see, everything Lance does, he takes seriously. He pours his heart and soul into every project and every person he encounters. Lance is a man of his word. He is compassionate, and persistent, and has a true desire to improve the world we live in.

So, it's no wonder that Lance is also a writer, author, influencer, and healthcare professional with over 20 years in the healthcare industry. He is known as a thought leader and inspiration to families and professionals around the world. Due to his desire to serve, he has received many awards:

- Lance was chosen as a "50 Under 50" for 2023 by the New York City Journal.

- Lance received The Silver Creator YouTube Award

- His Podcast All Home Care Matters is in the top .5% of all podcasts.

- Lance was chosen as a Juror for the Academy of Interactive Visual Arts for 2023.

In college, Lance was selected as one of only 70 college students nationally to study medicine in the People's Republic of China as a special medical delegation.

He was Named a Difference Maker at the University of Michigan - Dearborn. This prestigious honor is only awarded to the best of the best at Michigan.

Lance also writes monthly columns for some of the most prestigious publications in the healthcare industry:

- McKnight's Home Care News

- DailyCaring.com

- AgeBuzz

So far, I've just told you about Lance as a professional, but his personal life is just as impressive. Lance gave up his dream of being a doctor to care for his father when he became ill, caring for him in his own home with his wife. This experience was life-changing for Lance, and he still holds this moment in time close to his heart and is filled with gratitude for what he was taught and what he can now share with others.

Like most of you picking up this book, you probably feel lost, overwhelmed, and alone in a maze of medical confusion, jargon, and a new role that no one ever talked about let alone trained you for. That is exactly why you've been guided to read this step-by-step official family caregiver's guide.

Lance knows what it's like to not know what questions to ask or who to reach out to. His personal experience caring for a loved one combined with his professional knowledge of helping thousands of families will help you avoid the pitfalls and frustration common on this caregiving journey.

Lance is a family man. He is happily married with three children, who he coaches, supports, and makes sure they have their family movie nights on Fridays. He is a religious man who is extremely active in his church. He believes in having strong relationships with his children and sets high standards as their role model. He recently took on the role of Athletic Director on top of his regular job, at his children's school. To be honest, I don't know how he does all he does, but what I do know is he is driven to help people and make the world a better place.

I believe you will find his book to be your caregiving bible. One of those books you hang onto, that you make notes in, and tag pages you will want to reference many times. I believe you will not only find wonderful insights and guidance from Lance but also comfort in his words which will empower you through the good and bad days ahead. I believe you, like Lance will find gratitude in the many gifts you will receive as you care for another.

Honestly, I can say I've never heard a person say a negative word about Lance. Only praise for his kindness, and his openness to help others when in need without asking for a thing in return.

So, I encourage you to write a review for Lance's book or just drop him a note on how The All Home Care Matters Official Family Caregivers' Guide has helped you.

The man deserves a pat on the back for all he does for others. I know it will mean the world to him although he would never ask. Plus, I believe it will encourage him to write more. My guess is Lance has many more books in him, just waiting to come out.

Lance, I can't wait to see what you do next and I know I won't be the only one watching you!

In gratitude for all you do Lance -

Lori La Bey, founder of Alzheimer's Speaks

Table of Contents

Introduction:
The Dawn of Caregiving

Caregiving comes to us often subtly, quietly slipping into our daily routines as we watch our parents age. It's a natural progression that many face but are seldom prepared for. This crucial transition, when children gradually become caretakers, is filled with both poignant moments and significant challenges. At the very essence of this journey is the need to equip ourselves with knowledge, resources, and the emotional resilience to manage the welfare of those who once so lovingly cared for us. In this introductory chapter, we lay the foundation for understanding the multifaceted responsibilities that lie ahead and embrace the delicate balance of providing care while maintaining respect and nurturing independence.

As we approach this new chapter in our lives, it's imperative to recognize the early signs that our parents might need assistance and to establish open channels of communication. To do this, we must develop a compassionate yet practical mindset. You may find yourself in a role you never anticipated, requiring skills you never knew you possessed or needed. Here, at the dawn of caregiving, we begin our exploration into this uncharted territory with a sensitivity to the nuances and complexities of this life stage. We reflect on the responsibilities and the emotional dimensions that come with this new territory—preparing ourselves to act with foresight, love, and a well-informed perspective.

Transitioning into the role of a caregiver isn't merely about managing the day-to-day; it's about transforming our relationships,

1

expectations, and plans for the future. This introduction doesn't delve into the specific legal, medical, or financial tasks—that detailed guidance will come later. Instead, it's here to affirm that the feelings you're experiencing are both valid and shared by many. Our aim is to pave the way for the subsequent chapters that will serve as a roadmap, guiding you through the complexities of caregiving. So let's begin this journey together, with patience and understanding, as we navigate the dawn of caregiving—a time filled with both challenges and opportunities to deepen the bonds of love and care.

Chapter 1:
Recognizing the Shifts

As the dawn of caregiving transitions into the light of day, it becomes clear that our roles with our aging parents are changing. With each visit or phone call, we might begin to notice small, yet significant shifts in their abilities, behaviors, or circumstances. These nuances aren't rife with warning sirens; they more often whisper of a need for subtle adjustments or support. It's in the missed appointments or the cluttered home, once meticulously kept, that we may find the early signs that our parents require assistance. It's a delicate time—filled with nuance and requiring a keen, compassionate eye. Starting the conversation about these changes is not about jumping to conclusions but rather about acknowledging the evolution of their needs. It's the foundation upon which we'll build our understanding and approach to caregiving, always with the respect and love that our parents deserve. As we begin this journey together, let's gently explore, recognize, and prepare for the shifts that life inevitably brings.

Early Signs of Needing Assistance

As we navigate the ever-changing landscape of our parents' lives, vigilance becomes a subtle yet significant part of our routine. The process of understanding when your elderly parents might need help isn't always straightforward. Life's natural progression often masks itself in small changes, changes that, when pieced together, depict a larger shift requiring our attention.

One of the most telling signs that assistance may be needed is a noticeable decline in personal hygiene. This does not mean a skipped shower or two, but rather a consistent lack of grooming that is out of character for your parent. If you notice unkempt hair, a disregard for dental hygiene, or a significant deviation from their typical standards of cleanliness, it's time to consider a conversation about support.

Another indicator can be found in the home environment. A once tidy and well-maintained space becoming cluttered or dirty is a cause for concern. It may start small, with unwashed dishes piling up or laundry going undone, but these tasks can become increasingly difficult for aging parents to manage, signaling a need for assistance.

Additionally, take note of your parent's eating habits. Changes in weight, an empty fridge, or spoiled food can suggest difficulties in meal preparation or a loss of appetite. This shift might be due to physical challenges or decreased cognitive function, both warranting further exploration and support.

Pay attention to how your parents are managing their finances. Are bills being paid on time? Are there unopened pieces of mail stacking up? These could be early warning signs of cognitive decline or an inability to keep track of important tasks.

It's also important to monitor any changes in mobility. A sudden hesitation to walk, climb stairs, or fear of leaving the house can indicate underlying health issues. Mobility challenges not only limit independence but also increase the risk of falls and accidents at home.

On the topic of health, keep an eye out for medication management. Missing doses, confusion about prescriptions, or a lack of refills can have serious implications on your parents' health and are clear indications that intervention may be necessary.

When it comes to social interactions, a sharp decrease in engagement or withdrawal from previously enjoyed activities can be a red flag. Social isolation can have detrimental effects on mental and emotional well-being and may point to other issues such as depression or mobility problems.

Subtle changes in communication patterns may also arise. If your parents are harder to reach by phone, seem less talkative, or are neglecting to return messages, these can be signs of either physical issues, like hearing loss, or cognitive changes that require support.

Furthermore, look out for safety concerns such as unexplained bruising or injuries that might suggest falls or accidents occurring without your knowledge. It's crucial to address these concerns swiftly to prevent more serious harm.

It's also common to observe a decline in driving skills. If you notice dents in the car, hear about close calls, or see a general uncertainty in driving, it might be time to have a talk about alternative modes of transportation to ensure their safety.

Another area to be mindful of involves decision-making abilities. Hesitance or poor choices in scenarios that previously would have been handled with ease might suggest a decline in cognitive abilities, necessitating a closer look and potential support.

Remember that these signs might not all present themselves at once. It's often a gradual process. Keeping a gentle but watchful eye is key to recognizing when to step in. It's all about balance—acknowledging growing limitations without underestimating the abilities and independence your parents still hold dear.

While surfacing these concerns is essential, it's just as critical to approach them with sensitivity. The realization that help is needed can be a tough pill to swallow for many, and your approach should be steeped in empathy and understanding, leading with love and respect for their independence.

Each of these signals, while subtle on their own, may collectively indicate that it's time to consider what assistance your parents might need. The next step involves starting a thoughtful and candid conversation about these shifts, setting the stage for collaboration and planning that respects their autonomy and well-being.

Starting the Conversation

If you're noticing that your parents are beginning to need a bit more assistance, one of the most delicate steps is initiating the conversation about their care. It's often fraught with emotion and resistance, but it's an essential starting point on your caregiving journey. Acknowledging this isn't easy, but let's explore how you can approach this talk with compassion and clarity.

Firstly, choose the right time and place. It should be somewhere private, away from distractions, and at a time when none of you are feeling rushed. This creates a calm environment that is conducive to open and honest discussion.

Before you start, it's crucial to check your expectations at the door. Go into the conversation with an open mind and be ready to listen as much as you talk. Keep in mind that the goal is not to solve everything in one sitting but to start a dialogue.

Begin with expressing your observations without making assumptions. Mention specific incidents that have caused you concern. For instance, "I noticed you've been having trouble with the stairs" is better than saying, "You can't handle the stairs anymore."

As you share your concerns, take a collaborative tone. Use 'we' statements, like "How can we help make things safer for you?" This fosters a sense of teamwork and keeps the conversation from feeling adversarial.

It's equally important to be patient and give them time to absorb what's being said. They might be hearing their independence is waning for the first time, which can be tough to accept. Let them express their feelings and thoughts without interruption.

During this discussion, focus on the positives. Talk about how some changes could improve their quality of life. Maybe it's about having more leisure time or not having to deal with the stress of home maintenance.

Another aspect to consider is involving your parent in the decision-making process. Asking questions like "What do you feel you need help with?" can make them feel respected and in control. It's their life, and they need to be at the center of all decisions.

Be prepared for some resistance. It's natural for them to be skeptical or defensive. If they're not ready to talk about it, don't force the conversation. You can always revisit it later.

Remember, it's okay to involve other family members, but be careful about how many people join the conversation. Too many voices at once can be overwhelming. Decide on who your parent is most comfortable with and who can stay calm and constructive throughout the discussion.

Encourage your parent to share their wishes for the future. Do they have specific thoughts about where they would like to live or how they would like to receive care? This can guide planning and make them feel their desires are valued.

Demonstrate empathy and validation throughout the process. If your parent feels understood, they are more likely to be receptive to the conversation. Statements like "I understand this might be difficult to think about, but we want to make sure you're cared for" can go a long way.

Lastly, don't expect to cover all grounds in the first conversation. It's an ongoing discussion that evolves as needs change. What's essential is that the lines of communication are now open.

When the conversation ends, make sure everyone knows the next steps. Perhaps it's gathering more information, talking to professionals, or scheduling follow-up conversations. Clear action items can help clarify what's expected from each person involved.

Concluding this conversation on a positive note is as significant as starting it. Reiteration of your love and support can do wonders to ease tensions that may have risen during the chat. It's a delicate transition for everyone involved, and compassion, patience, and understanding are the keys to navigating it successfully.

Chapter 2:
The Basics of Caregiving

As you navigate the inevitable changes that accompany your parents' aging process, understanding the fundamentals of caregiving becomes a cornerstone of providing effective support. It's about balancing compassion with practicality, where you learn to recognize when your presence is needed for more than just companionship—when you become a crucial part of your loved one's daily life. Accepting your new role can be as much about managing your expectations as it is about providing care. It's a journey where patience must intertwine with decisive action, and the lines of communication between you and your parents need to remain as open as ever. In this chapter, we'll focus on the core aspects of caregiving, including defining what your role entails and how to set realistic goals for yourself and the ones you care for. It's important to remind yourself that you're not alone; many have walked this path, and with the right approach, you'll find a balance that respects both your needs and those of your aging parents.

Understanding Your Role

In embarking upon the caregiving journey, it's vital to have a clear understanding of what the role entitles. Caregiving is a multifaceted responsibility, one that evolves and adapts to the needs of your aging parent. As you transition into this new phase, you'll find that the position demands emotional support, managerial skills, and unwavering patience.

Firstly, you must identify what your parent requires from you. Do they need help managing medications, assistance with daily activities, or simply a listening ear? Each scenario requires a different approach. By assessing their needs effectively, you can prepare to fulfill your role in a way that suits both you and your parent.

A crucial aspect of understanding your role is recognizing the boundaries of your abilities. You're stepping into this out of love and concern, but you are not a professional healthcare provider. It's essential to ascertain when to seek help and whom to consult for various types of care and advice. Trying to do everything yourself is neither sustainable nor advisable.

Communication is the cornerstone of your caregiving role. Developing an open dialogue with your parent allows you to respect their wishes and maintain their dignity. Remember that while you may be the caregiver, your parent is still an adult with their own preferences and autonomy.

It's equally important to establish clear and open communication with other family members who may share the responsibility with you. Whether providing moral support, physical help, or financial assistance, every family member must be on the same page about care strategies and objectives.

An often-overlooked element of caregiving is the sheer amount of coordination involved. You'll likely find yourself juggling appointments, medication schedules, and daily routines. Staying organized is not just about convenience; it's critical for ensuring that nothing vital is overlooked in your parent's care.

Compassion comes naturally to most when caring for a loved one, but it's necessary to be mindful of the empathy fatigue that can envelop you. Recognizing the emotional toll this role can take will arm you with the mindfulness needed to seek support when the burden feels too heavy.

Another component of your role is being an advocate for your parent. As they age, they may encounter more complex health issues and a less robust ability to challenge or question healthcare providers. You'll often find yourself in situations where you need to stand up for their best interests, whether it's in a medical, legal, or personal context.

Adaptability is key. As time progresses, your parent's needs will change, sometimes unexpectedly. Being prepared to adjust your caregiving approach at a moment's notice is part of the territory.

Financial oversight may fall to you as well. This could involve anything from balancing a checkbook to managing insurance claims or medical bills. Approach these tasks with accuracy and honesty to maintain financial stability and trust.

Moreover, integral to your role is the ongoing education about your parent's medical conditions and the aging process. This knowledge is power – it helps in making informed decisions and discussions with healthcare providers more impactful.

Don't underestimate the role of self-care in your new position. Managing your own health and well-being affects your ability to provide care. If you neglect this aspect, you risk burnout and being unable to care for your parent effectively.

Finally, your role as a caregiver may include preparing for the inevitability of tough conversations and decisions. Whether discussing living arrangements, end-of-life wishes, or the need for additional help, approach these dialogues with sensitivity and respect for their feelings and opinions.

Remember, your role is dynamic and deeply personal. It's crafted from your unique relationship with your parent and the specific needs that arise from their situation. Balancing pragmatism with sensitivity will make you an effective caregiver who serves with heart and integrity.

In closing this section, it's paramount to acknowledge that this role, like any other with great responsibility, is learned and perfected over time. Be patient with yourself and open to learning from each experience. The fact that you've undertaken this role speaks volumes about your love and commitment. Hold on to that as you navigate the intricacies of caregiving.

Setting Realistic Expectations

As you step into the role of caregiver, understanding the importance of setting realistic expectations cannot be overstated. This isn't just about aligning your goals with what's achievable—it's also about protecting your own well-being throughout this process. Let's face it: caring for an aging parent is not only physically demanding but also emotionally complex. You're navigating a new dynamic in your relationship, filled with changes that you might not feel prepared for.

First, assess what you can reasonably do with the time and resources you have. You might want to do everything for your parent, but it's important to acknowledge that you have limitations. Whether it's time constraints due to work or other responsibilities, physical limitations, or a lack of specific expertise in medical or legal matters, recognizing these boundaries early will help avoid feelings of failure or guilt down the line.

Secondly, discuss expectations with your parent. They may have their own ideas of what they need and what you can provide. It's crucial to have open and honest conversations about what's possible and make adjustments together. Bear in mind, your parent may be dealing with feelings of loss of independence and may struggle to accept help, which is why maintaining a dialogue is key to understanding each other's perspectives.

Consider the tasks that need to be addressed. Caregiving involves a myriad of responsibilities that can range from simple companionship to complex medical care. Evaluate which tasks you can handle on your own and those that you might need help with, whether from other family members, friends, or professional services. This will not only help set a practical caregiving plan in motion but also help you delineate clear boundaries for yourself.

Setting a realistic care plan also involves understanding that certain aspects of your parent's health and capabilities may fluctuate. The level and type of care needed can change unexpectedly, and it's imperative to stay adaptable. Just as youth is marked by growth, aging is marked by change—sometimes gradual, sometimes sudden. Be prepared for both.

Understandably, you might feel obligated to meet every need your parent has, but it's vital to accept that some days will be better than others. Some tasks will be carried out seamlessly, while others might be left undone. That's not a reflection of inadequacy; it's just the nature of life and caregiving.

Furthermore, it's important to temper your expectations regarding improvements or reversals in your parent's condition. Aging is a natural process, and while certain interventions can enhance quality of life, expecting things to return to how they were years ago can lead to disappointment. Appreciate the small victories and focus on making today as good as it can be.

There's also a financial reality to consider. You may need to invest in modifications to your parent's home or in-home care services, or even consider the eventual move to an assisted living facility. Being realistic about what you can afford will guide decisions and avoid financial strain in the future.

It's also essential to set realistic expectations with your own family and employer. Caregiving can impact your availability and energy levels, so communicating with your spouse, children, or supervisor can ensure they understand your new responsibilities and can provide support when necessary.

Remember to factor in self-care. Just as flight attendants instruct passengers to put on their own oxygen mask before helping others, you must take care of your well-being to be an effective caregiver. If you're depleted, you won't be able to provide the level of care your parent needs. Realistically, this might mean scheduling time away from caregiving duties to recharge.

Be realistic about the emotional toll as well. Watching a parent age and become more dependent can stir a range of emotions, from sadness to frustration. It's natural to feel this way, but expecting to manage everything with constant grace is setting yourself up for disappointment. Seek out support groups or a therapist who can help manage these complex feelings.

Set milestones and adjust as necessary. In your caregiving journey, you might set goals related to your parent's health or your ability to balance responsibilities. Recognize that these goals may need to be adjusted. What's important is that you're making progress and reassessing as you go along.

Accepting help is also part of setting realistic expectations. You can't do it all alone, and accepting help isn't a sign of weakness—it's a practical step. Look into local resources, professional caregivers, or technology that can assist in your caregiving tasks. Leverage the help available to create a sustainable support system for both you and your parent.

Lastly, embody patience. Change doesn't occur overnight, and neither does adapting to the role of caregiver. You'll learn, grow, and find your rhythm in time. Patience with yourself, your parent, and the situation as a whole will go a long way in maintaining your resilience throughout this journey.

Caregiving is complex and multifaceted, but by setting realistic expectations, you anchor yourself and your parent in a situation that is manageable. Embrace the role with compassion and pragmatism, knowing that you're doing your utmost within the limits of what's possible. This grounded approach will not only provide your parent with the best care you can offer but will also preserve your own well-being in the long run.

Chapter 3:
Legal and Financial Planning

As the caregiving journey unfolds, securing your parents' legal and financial matters becomes imperative. Tackling these issues early can prevent unnecessary stress and complications down the road. It's about understanding not just what essential documents you'll need, but also how to navigate the complex waters of insurance and benefits, which sometimes feel like they're written in a foreign language. In this chapter, we'll delve into creating a solid legal foundation, ensuring that all necessary paperwork, from powers of attorney to living wills, is in place and up to date. We'll demystify financial planning for long-term care, addressing how to weave through the Medicare maze and seize every benefit available to your parents. Embarking on this path now can spare you from daunting legal battles or financial crises in the future, allowing you to focus on what matters most—caring for your loved ones with peace of mind.

Essential Documents

As you embark on the journey of caregiving for your aging parents, one of the most crucial steps is ensuring that all essential legal and financial documents are in place. This isn't just about ticking boxes; it's about peace of mind, preparedness, and ensuring that your loved ones' wishes are honored. These documents form the cornerstone of effective legal and financial planning, and they safeguard both you and your parents from potential future uncertainties.

Let's begin with the basics: the power of attorney (POA). A POA allows your parent to designate someone to make decisions on their behalf should they become unable to do so. This can include handling financial matters, such as paying bills or managing investments, or making health care decisions if they are not in a position to express their wishes. It's critical to discuss this with your parents early on to understand their preferences and to appoint someone they trust implicitly.

A living will, meanwhile, is a document that outlines your parents' wishes regarding life-sustaining treatment in the event they are incapacitated and unable to communicate. This can include directives about the use of resuscitation, mechanical ventilation, or feeding tubes. It's a delicate conversation, but it's better to have their wishes captured when they're able to express them knowingly and willfully.

Advance directives are closely related to living wills but cover a broader array of decisions. Besides medical treatment, these directives can address pain management, organ donation, and end-of-life care. Often included with a living will and medical power of attorney, an advance directive ensures that health care providers and loved ones are clear on your parents' preferences.

It's important to remember that these documents aren't just forms to be filled out and forgotten. They represent your parents' autonomy and should be crafted carefully, with thoughtful consideration of all the possible scenarios they may face. Consulting with an attorney who specializes in elder law can help in tailoring these documents to your family's specific needs and state laws.

Moving onto financial planning, it's essential to have a list of accounts, policies, and assets, alongside the appropriate documentation. This includes but is not limited to bank accounts, retirement accounts, life insurance policies, real estate deeds, and personal property documentation. Knowing where these are kept, and ensuring they are easily accessible in an organized manner, will remove much of the stress and confusion that can accompany financial matters in times of crisis.

Another key document is the HIPAA release form. This form grants others permission to access your parents' private health information. Without this, you may find yourself unable to get necessary updates or make informed decisions about their healthcare needs.

While it's natural to hesitate when facing these topics—they confront the very real and sometimes uncomfortable themes of vulnerability and mortality—it's also an act of love and responsibility. It paves the way for open discussion between you and your parents about their wishes, hopes, and expectations. Plus, addressing these matters proactively allows for a smoother transition should the documents ever need to be enacted.

You'll also want to consider drafting a list of all debts, including mortgages, car loans, and credit cards. Understanding the liabilities your parents have is just as critical as knowing their assets. This aids in managing their financial landscape and preventing any unwelcome surprises along the journey.

When these documents are complete, it is not enough to just tuck them away in a safe deposit box and forget about them. It's important to review them periodically with your parents, making sure they still represent their current wishes and updating them as necessary. Laws change, as do individual circumstances, so regular review is essential.

Moreover, make sure key family members know where these documents are stored and that they can access them when needed. This includes ensuring that all designated decision-makers have copies or know where to obtain copies quickly, in the event of an emergency or urgent decision-making situation.

It's also beneficial to have a list of your parents' advisors and contacts, including their attorney, accountant, financial planner, and insurance agents. In a circumstance where you need to make decisions or gather information on their behalf, you'll know exactly who to turn to.

Remember that while it's important to honor the spirit of your parents' wishes, the letter of the law will govern. Each state has its own specific requirements for how these documents must be executed to be legally binding. For instance, some states require notarization while others may require witnesses, and sometimes both. Therefore, seek guidance to ensure everything is in order based on your particular location.

Finally, resist the temptation to speed through these conversations with your parents. Take the time to listen to their concerns and understand their values. The process of securing these essential documents often provides richness in connection, allowing for deep and meaningful conversations about life, the care they hope to receive, and their legacy.

With all these steps attended to, you can approach the care of your aging parents with the assurance that their legal and financial matters are safeguarded. This documentation backbones the planning, but it's woven with the threads of empathy, respect, and foresight. Approaching it with the necessary gravity and thoroughness will ensure that no matter what lies ahead, you and your parents are as prepared as possible.

Navigating Insurance and Benefits

The journey into the world of insurance and benefits for an aging parent is much like a labyrinth; it's intricate, complex, and requires patient navigation. As you assume this facet of their care, understanding the nuances of various policies and programs becomes vital. In this section, we'll explore the key elements of insurance and benefits that you need to tackle to secure your parent's welfare as they age.

Firstly, it's crucial to get a comprehensive overview of your parent's insurance policies. This includes not only health insurance but also life, long-term care, and any supplemental insurance they may have. Ensure you have access to all policy documents and understand the coverage details and any associated costs such as premiums, deductibles, copayments, and coinsurance.

When it comes to health insurance, Medicare often takes center stage for those over 65 or with certain disabilities. Familiarize yourself with the different parts of Medicare: Part A covers hospital insurance, Part B provides medical insurance, Part C offers Medicare Advantage Plans, and Part D covers prescription drugs. Each part has its own enrollment periods and coverage specifications, which are pivotal in planning your parent's care.

Don't overlook the importance of Medicare Supplement Insurance, also known as Medigap. These policies can help cover costs that Medicare doesn't, such as copayments and deductibles. Each Medigap policy offers different levels of coverage and comes with its own set of policies, so comparing options is key to finding the right fit for your parent's needs.

Long-term care insurance is another aspect to delve into. If your parent has a policy, understand what it covers, like nursing home care or in-home care services. The specifics of how benefits are paid out— per day, per visit, or in a lump sum—can greatly affect how you plan for possible long-term care scenarios.

Life insurance policies can sometimes be a source of funds for care through accelerating death benefits or life settlements. These options can be complex and have tax implications, so consulting with a financial advisor or an insurance specialist is recommended to weigh the pros and cons.

For veterans, there may be benefits available through the Department of Veterans Affairs (VA) that can assist with healthcare and long-term care needs. If your parent served in the military, investigating these benefits could uncover valuable resources for their care plan.

Aside from these insurance considerations, it's also worth looking into benefit programs such as Social Security, which provides retirement and disability income, and Supplemental Security Income (SSI), which assists older adults with little to no income. These programs can form a critical part of your parent's financial stability.

Understanding your parent's employer-provided benefits, both past and present, can uncover continuing health care options or life insurance benefits. Pensions or retirement plans from past employment should also be reviewed to grasp their impact on your parent's financial situation.

When managing these insurances and benefits, ensure that all premiums are paid on time to avoid lapses in coverage. Automating payments or setting up reminders can help manage these critical tasks amidst a potentially busy caregiving schedule.

Being well-informed about your parent's health condition is crucial when dealing with insurance. Certain policies may have specific stipulations or exclusions based on pre-existing conditions, and knowing these in detail can prevent unexpected expenses.

Moreover, knowing the deadlines for enrollment periods and claims submission is imperative. Medicare, for instance, has strict enrollment periods which, if missed, can lead to penalties or delayed coverage. Similarly, insurance claims have filing deadlines which, if missed, can result in out-of-pocket expenses.

Claims processing and paperwork can be daunting. Make sure to thoroughly document every medical visit, procedure, and prescription. This will ease the submission of claims and ensure that your parent receives all the benefits they're entitled to. Should disputes with insurance providers arise, meticulous records will be your best defense.

For times when you're unsure of the specifics or need personalized advice, don't hesitate to contact insurance agents, benefit coordinators, or a trusted elder law attorney. Over the phone consults or face-to-face meetings can provide clarity and guidance in interpreting the sometimes complex language of policies.

Finally, as health needs evolve, so too might insurance and benefit requirements. Regularly review your parent's coverage to ensure it keeps pace with their changing needs. Adjusting policies or benefits may be necessary to provide the most cost-effective and comprehensive care for your parent.

Charting a path through the insurance and benefits landscape requires patience, attention to detail, and a proactive approach. Your diligence in navigating these waters will help ensure that your aging parent's health and financial needs are well-protected, enhancing their quality of life as they transition into this next stage.

Chapter 4:
The Emotional Journey

As you've familiarized yourself with the legal and financial foundation of caregiving, you're likely discovering that traversing the internal landscape is as crucial as managing the tangible aspects. The emotional journey of caring for your aging parents isn't something you can neatly plot on a graph or to-do list; it's a roller coaster with unexpected twists, deep dives, and, occasionally, moments of profound grace. It's normal to feel a complex mosaic of emotions— from guilt over feeling burdened to grief as you watch them decline. Much of the challenge lies in the role reversal that takes place, as you shift from being the cared-for to the caregiver. The resilience you'll need isn't just about pushing through; it's about allowing yourself to feel vulnerable, acknowledging the depth of your emotions, and finding strength in your compassion. This chapter will walk through navigating your own feelings, as well as addressing the emotions that might come up for your parents, including their possible resistance or denial of the need for help. It's pivotal to remember you're not alone; countless others have walked this path, paving the way with insights that can illuminate your own journey.

Coping with Role Reversal

Caring for aging parents often comes with subtle beginnings – an extra reminder here, a hand with bills there. Before you know it, this shift crests into a full role reversal where you, the child, find yourself in the caregiver position. It's a phase of life that you might anticipate, but the emotional complexity only becomes clear as you face it directly.

Coping with this turnabout means acknowledging a spectrum of emotions. You might grapple with feelings of sadness as you witness your parents' decline, or frustration at the increased demands on your time. Compassion and concern can quickly mesh with resentment and guilt, all normal in this rearrangement of family dynamics.

Understanding that this role reversal is a part of the natural cycle of life can be comforting. It allows you to see the situation with perspective and approach your new responsibilities with grace. Remembering the care your parents once provided you, in whatever form that took, can also create a bridge to acceptance.

Starting this new chapter requires clear communication. It's essential to speak openly with your parents about the changes that are occurring. Establishing this dialogue early on can help prevent misunderstandings and pave the way for cooperative decision-making. It's also a means to gauge their comfort levels and respect their autonomy as much as possible.

Boundaries need to be set to balance the new caregiving duties with your own life. Overstepping can lead to burnout and strain relationships. Therefore, determine what you can feasibly handle and find support for the areas where you can't. This could mean involving other family members or looking into professional caregiving services.

It's natural to wrestle with guilt, often feeling like you're not doing enough. Remember, caregiving is not about perfection; it's about providing love and support to the best of your ability. Accepting that you have limitations is a step towards emotional well-being and better care for your parents.

Maintaining a sense of your parents' identity, and your own, outside of the caregiver relationship is vital. Encourage their hobbies and interests, ensuring they continue to live a life filled with purpose and joy. At the same time, make sure to keep up with your own activities and interests. This division helps keep resentment at bay.

Seeking out resources can make a world of difference. Whether it's a caregiver support group or utilizing respite services, these resources can offer emotional relief and practical assistance. They can be a haven for sharing experiences and discovering coping strategies from those traveling a similar road.

The legal and financial aspect of role reversal also introduces its own set of challenges. Tackling these early on and head-on, as covered in Chapter 3, can alleviate many potential stressors later down the road. Having essential documents in place and understanding the ins and outs of insurance and benefits will bring peace of mind.

It's crucial to practice compassion, for your parents and yourself. In moments of conflict or stress, take a step back and try to view the situation through the lens of empathy. Forgiving yourself and your parents when things don't go as planned is a form of self-care that benefits everyone involved.

As you navigate these new waters, remember that change is constant. Flexibility will be your ally as your parents' needs evolve and as you evolve alongside them. While your roles may have shifted, the essence of your relationship – love and mutual respect – remains the same.

Don't shy away from professional advice when needed. Whether it's a counselor to help address the emotional labor or a care manager to assist in coordinating the various aspects of caregiving, external expertise can provide a clearer path forward.

Preparing for the days ahead means acknowledging that there may come a time when caring at home is no longer the best option. This preparation, as portrayed in Chapter 7, sets the stage for the possibility of transitioning to assisted living. Having these potential plans in place can reduce anxiety for everyone involved.

In moments of doubt or overwhelm, remind yourself that you are not alone in this journey. Millions are walking the path of caregiving, facing the same dilemmas, the same poignant transformations. They too are learning how to balance the past with the present, the giving with receiving, the child with the adult.

Ultimately, coping with role reversal is about love – adapting to express it in its new form. It's about nurturing the bonds that have tied you together through the years and finding new ways to strengthen them as the caregiving journey unfolds.

Dealing with Resistance and Denial

When you're navigating the emotional journey of caregiving, one of the most challenging hurdles can be dealing with your aging parents' resistance and denial about their changing needs. Acceptance doesn't always come easily, especially when it involves loss of independence. Understanding the roots of this resistance is a critical starting point in addressing it.

Often, the resistance you encounter is born from a deep sense of fear and loss. Your parents may fear losing their autonomy, the comfort of familiar routines, and the very home they've perhaps lived in for decades. They may also be in denial about their situation. It's important to approach these conversations with sensitivity and patience.

When confronting denial, it's crucial to remember that your parents may truly not see the signs of decline that you're noticing. The gradual nature of aging can sometimes make changes less obvious to the person experiencing them. To help them see your perspective, provide specific, tangible examples of your concerns instead of vague observations.

As you broach this topic, try to engage in a dialogue rather than a monologue. Ask open-ended questions that encourage your parents to express their feelings and fears. This can create a more collaborative environment where you're working together to find solutions rather than dictating what needs to be done.

It's also helpful to have these conversations in a neutral, comfortable setting where your parents don't feel cornered. A place where they feel at ease may lead to a more open exchange of thoughts. Remember to speak with respect and avoid patronizing language that could make them feel belittled or infantilized.

Expect that you may need to have multiple conversations. Resistance and denial aren't typically conquered in a single discussion. Be prepared to have a gradual, layered conversation that develops over time, allowing your parents to process the information and their emotions at a pace they can handle.

Another effective strategy can be involving an unbiased third party, such as a doctor, geriatric care manager, or a close family friend your parents trust. Sometimes hearing concerns from someone who isn't directly involved in the day-to-day can make the reality easier to accept.

When your parents are in denial about their need for assistance, consider focusing on the benefits of the help rather than the help itself. You might illustrate how certain services or adjustments could enhance their independence, rather than reduce it. For instance, hiring a cleaning service can be framed as a way to save energy for more enjoyable activities.

In some cases, small steps can be a way to ease into larger changes. Starting with a minimal level of assistance, like having a professional come in once a week to help with household tasks, allows your parents to gradually become accustomed to receiving help and realizing its benefits.

However, if resistance persists and is jeopardizing their safety or health, it may be necessary to be more assertive. You still need to express empathy for their situation, but also convey the seriousness of your concerns. It's a delicate balance between respect for their autonomy and your responsibility as a caregiver to ensure their well-being.

Self-care is vital during this process, as resistance and denial can be emotionally taxing for you as a caregiver. Take time for yourself to decompress and seek support from other caregivers who understand the challenges you face. Remember that you're not alone in this and others have navigated these choppy waters too.

Documenting your observations and their responses can be helpful, especially when you need to recall earlier conversations or make decisions. Keeping notes can also assist in tracking any progression in their condition or in the effectiveness of the strategies you're employing.

One thing to always avoid is an argumentative tone, as it rarely leads to constructive outcomes. Aim for empathic listening and try to validate their emotions, even when you're pushing for important changes. Remember that you're both on the same team, aiming for the best quality of life possible.

Finally, be willing to adjust your approach as needed. If one method isn't working, try another. The key is to stay flexible and creative in your problem-solving. Resistance and denial may be part of your caregiving journey, but with patience, understanding, and tenacity, you can navigate these challenges effectively.

Dealing with resistance and denial is never easy, but it's a natural part of the emotional journey in caregiving. By approaching your aging parents with compassion, involving them in the process, and incrementally introducing assistance, you can help them maintain their dignity and sense of control during the transitions ahead.

Chapter 5:
Health and Medical Needs

Tending to the health and medical needs of our aging parents can be one of the most complex aspects of caregiving. It's a delicate balance of empowering their independence and stepping in when necessary. This chapter has been tailored to guide you through the nuances of routine health management—ensuring that both the everyday and the critical medical needs of your loved ones are met with understanding and efficiency. As you navigate this chapter, you'll learn how to keep regular health checks on track, the importance of medication management, and how to stay alert for signs that additional medical support might be needed. You'll also gain insights into identifying potential emergencies quickly and how to respond effectively. Remember, maintaining open lines of communication with healthcare providers and staying informed are key to managing the complexities of your parents' health—a journey that requires patience, vigilance, and the knowledge that this guide aims to offer.

Routine Health Management

As we embrace the responsibility of caring for our aging parents, understanding the nuances of routine health management becomes paramount. This facet of their well-being is as crucial as any emergency that might arise. However, routine care is preventative, aiming to maintain a stable and comfortable quality of life for as long as possible.

One of the first steps in managing our parents' health is to create a comprehensive list of their current medical conditions and medications. This list should include dosages, frequency, and the purpose of each medication. It's wise to review this list periodically with their healthcare provider to ensure efficacy and to make adjustments as necessary.

Another aspect of routine health management is scheduling regular check-ups and screenings. These visits to the doctor are vital in catching potential issues early. Discussions with healthcare providers during these visits should go beyond the immediate concerns and encompass lifestyle, diet, exercise, and any changes in mental health.

Monitoring your parents' diet is a core component of their health. An appropriate, nutritious diet can be the key to managing chronic illnesses, maintaining energy levels, and improving mood. Consulting a dietician if needed, and possibly meal planning services, can ensure that dietary needs are being addressed.

Physical activity, as advised by a healthcare professional, is essential. Encourage your parents to engage in exercise, whether it's a daily walk, senior yoga classes, or other activities they enjoy. Physical activity not only supports physical health but also mental well-being.

Preserving mental health is just as important as physical health. If you notice changes in mood, memory, or behavior, it's important to discuss these with a healthcare professional. Staying mentally active with puzzles, reading, and social activities can support cognitive function.

Medication adherence is a common issue among the elderly. Setting up a system, such as a weekly pill organizer or using a medication management service, can help ensure that medications are taken correctly and at the right times.

It's also worth considering the use of technology to aid in health management. There are various apps and devices designed to track health metrics, remind about medication, and even connect directly with healthcare providers.

Sleep is a critical element of health that often gets overlooked. Maintaining a regular sleep pattern can have a positive impact on overall health. Encourage and help create an environment that is conducive to good sleep, such as a cool, dark, and quiet room.

Vision and hearing are senses that commonly decline with age. Make sure your parents have regular vision and hearing checks, and address any issues with glasses or hearing aids promptly to maintain their quality of life.

Dental health shouldn't fall by the wayside either. Oral health issues can lead to other health problems, so regular dental check-ups and daily care are important.

Managing your parents' healthcare appointments can be overwhelming. Creating a calendar with reminders for appointments, prescription refills, and routine screenings can help you stay organized.

Understanding your parents' health insurance coverage is critical to managing their routine care. Being aware of what services and medications are covered and which healthcare providers are within the network can prevent unexpected expenses.

In the event that your parent must be admitted to a hospital, it's important to have a hospital bag prepared. This bag can include items like their insurance information, a list of medications, and any personal items they may need. Quick access to this information is essential for healthcare providers and can ease the stress of an unplanned hospital visit.

Lastly, the most important aspect of routine health management is communication. Open, honest discussions with your aging parents about their health and preferences can help you make informed decisions together. It's about empowering them to maintain their independence and dignity while ensuring their safety and health are not compromised.

In these paragraphs, we've woven together a tapestry of considerations that, when addressed diligently, can lay a solid foundation for managing the routine health of our loved ones. Each element serves a distinct purpose in upholding their best potential quality of life, highlighting our commitment and love as we navigate this heartfelt journey.

Recognizing and Responding to Medical Emergencies

As you navigate the responsibilities of caring for an aging parent, being able to identify and correctly respond to medical emergencies is of utmost importance. Emergencies can happen suddenly, and knowing the steps to take can be the difference between life and death. It's a heavy burden to bear, but being prepared can ease some of that weight.

First and foremost, it's crucial to understand what constitutes a medical emergency. Signs such as chest pain, difficulty breathing, sudden confusion, or severe, uncontrolled bleeding are clear indicators that immediate medical attention is needed. If your parent experiences a fall resulting in loss of consciousness or an inability to get up, this too requires urgent care.

When faced with an emergency, your response should be swift and decisive. Begin by calling 911 and providing the dispatcher with all relevant information. Remain calm and clear while relaying the symptoms, as this helps paramedics prepare for the situation they'll be encountering. Remember, in these moments, you're the crucial link between your loved one and the medical professionals who can help them.

While waiting for help to arrive, your actions can greatly impact your parent's well-being. If they're conscious, use soothing words to reassure them. Try to collect any vital medical information that paramedics might need, like a list of current medications, allergies, and any known health conditions. This is where having a well-maintained and easily accessible list can be invaluable.

If your parent is unresponsive, check for breathing and a pulse. If they aren't breathing or you can't find a pulse, begin CPR if you've been trained to do so, and continue until help arrives. Having taken a CPR and emergency response course can make a critical difference here, and if you haven't yet, now is the time to consider it.

In the case of bleeding, apply direct pressure to the wound with a clean cloth to help stem the flow. Never attempt to move your parent unless they're in immediate danger, such as from fire or the risk of drowning. Instead, keep them as comfortable as possible and monitor their condition until the emergency services take over.

Remember, some emergencies aren't as visible as a fall or injury. For instance, strokes can present with subtle signs such as sudden weakness in one part of the body, difficulty speaking, or a drooping face. Act quickly if you notice these signs and remember the acronym "FAST" - Face, Arms, Speech, and Time. The faster a stroke is treated, the better the outcome may be.

In case of a seizure, keep your parent safe by clearing the area of anything hard or sharp. Place them on their side to help keep their airway clear. Don't try to restrain them or put anything in their mouth. Once the seizure passes, make them comfortable and speak to them in a comforting tone as they regain awareness.

It's also essential to consider the potential for medication-related emergencies. Incorrect dosages or interactions between different prescriptions can lead to serious issues. Be diligent about managing their medications and understand the possible side effects. In an emergency that might be medication-related, bring their medication list or the actual bottles for the emergency responders to review.

After an emergency, it's likely your parent will require follow-up care. Whether it's a hospital stay or additional appointments with specialists, ensure you're actively involved in understanding their treatment plan and the steps for recovery. Don't hesitate to ask questions and seek clarity about any instructions provided by healthcare professionals.

Dealing with a medical emergency is not just about the moment of crisis; it's also about the aftermath. Ensuring your home is a safe environment for recovery is part of your caregiving role. You might need to make adjustments like installing grab bars, using a hospital bed, or arranging for home health services.

Mental and emotional support is also pivotal during recovery. Your parent might feel vulnerable or scared after an emergency, and your reassurance can help alleviate those fears. Keep an open line of communication with them about their concerns and encourage them to express their feelings.

In the wake of an emergency, it's also time to assess or reassess your preparedness. Was there anything that could have been done differently? Are there additional warning signs or symptoms that you should now be aware of? Use this experience to update your knowledge and perhaps your emergency plans, too.

Finally, while caring for your parent, don't neglect your own emotional needs. Witnessing a loved one in a medical emergency can be a traumatic experience, and it's important to acknowledge the impact it may have on you. Seek support, whether through friends, a support group, or a professional counselor, to process your feelings and avoid caregiver burnout.

Preparing for medical emergencies is not about inviting pessimism into your caregiving journey; rather, it's about ensuring safety and poise in the face of unexpected challenges. With a prepared mind and compassionate heart, you'll be equipped to handle the pivotal role of protector as you guide your parent through their golden years.

Chapter 6:
At-Home Care Strategies

Transitioning into the role of an at-home caregiver demands a strategic and loving approach, especially when ensuring the safety and well-being of our aging parents in the familiarity of their own home. In this chapter, we'll explore practical methods for creating a secure environment that fosters both mobility and independence. Understanding how to organize effective home care is central to this strategy, allowing your loved ones to not only receive the support they need but also to maintain a sense of dignity and autonomy. We'll focus on establishing routines that suit their individual needs and adapting the household to prevent accidents while simplifying daily tasks. This process also involves selecting the right equipment and technological aids that can facilitate care without overwhelming the caregiver or the care receiver. By the end of this chapter, you'll be equipped with the knowledge to set up a compassionate and efficient at-home care system that is both empowering for your parents and manageable for you.

Safety and Mobility in the Home

Maintaining a safe and mobile environment in the home is paramount when caring for aging parents. It's a delicate balance, ensuring they can move freely while minimizing the risk of falls and accidents. Home is where your loved ones should feel most comfortable and secure, and with some thoughtful adjustments, you can significantly enhance their safety.

First and foremost, start with a thorough walk-through of your parent's living space. Identify potential tripping hazards such as loose rugs, electrical cords, and clutter. These should be addressed immediately—secure rugs with non-slip pads, manage cords with organizers, and clear clutter from walkways. It's also essential to ensure walkways are well-lit, so consider upgrading lighting in dimly lit areas.

Stairs can be a major challenge for the elderly. If your parents' home has multiple levels, assess whether they need additional support like handrails or stairlifts. If they're using mobility aids, make sure these devices can be used safely on the stairs. Sometimes the best course of action may be to arrange their living space so they can reside comfortably on one level.

Bathroom safety is crucial, as this area is a common site for falls. Install grab bars in the shower and near the toilet to provide support. Non-slip mats in the shower or bathtub can prevent slips, and a shower chair may be beneficial for those who have difficulty standing for extended periods.

In the kitchen, organize commonly used items to be within easy reach, reducing the need to climb on stools or bend excessively. This simple step can prevent falls and strain. If your parents have difficulty with grip strength, consider utensils and jar openers designed for easier handling.

For parents with compromised mobility, assess the feasibility of a personal emergency response system (PERS). This service provides a wearable call button, which can be a lifeline in the event of a fall or emergency. Knowing help is just a button push away can give both of you peace of mind.

Visually inspect the flooring throughout the home. Are there any loose floorboards or uneven tiles? Any irregularities need repair to present a uniform, stable surface. For homes with slippery surfaces, such as polished hardwood or tile, rugs with a non-slip underside can add traction.

Furniture arrangement can also impact safety and mobility. Ensure there is ample space to walk around furniture, and remove or reposition any pieces that obstruct a clear path. Moreover, sturdy furniture can sometimes serve as an interim support for balance, so keep this in mind while making adjustments.

In some cases, your parents might need assistive devices for mobility, like walkers or wheelchairs. It's imperative that these devices are not only the right fit for them but also compatible with their living environment. Doorway widths should be checked, and any necessary modifications should be made to accommodate them.

If cognitive decline is a factor, consider implementing more direct safety measures. This might include latches on cabinets that contain potentially harmful supplies or setting up alarms to alert you if your parents wander or leave the house unexpectedly.

Technology can play a role in enhancing home safety, too. Automatic shut-off features can be installed on appliances to prevent accidents, while smart home devices may help you control lighting, temperature, and locks remotely, keeping the environment safe and comfortable.

We mustn't ignore the outdoors when considering home safety. Ensure walkways are free from obstructions, well-maintained, and have good lighting. Repair any uneven paving, and during colder months, keep pathways clear of ice and snow.

Remember to discuss these changes with your parents. Involving them in the decision-making process not only empowers them but also helps to minimize resistance. Explain the reasons for each modification and how it will benefit their safety and independence. It's also important to check in regularly to see if their needs have changed or if further adjustments are necessary.

Finally, one of the least talked about aspects of safety is emergency preparedness. Make sure your parents' home has working smoke detectors, fire extinguishers, and a clear plan in case of emergencies. They should know where to go, whom to call, and have easy access to their important documents.

Securing the home against potential risks is a process that takes care, consideration, and ongoing attention. With each proactive step, you're not only safeguarding their well-being but also offering yourself reassurance that the place they call home is as safe as possible for them to enjoy their golden years. Remember, while these measures can seem overwhelming, they go a long way in preserving your parents' independence and quality of life.

Organizing Effective Home Care

When your parents begin to show signs that they need help with daily living, organizing effective home care becomes a pressing priority. This endeavor isn't just about hiring help or rearranging furniture; it's about creating a comprehensive plan that respects your parents' wishes and ensures their safety and well-being. In this section, we'll discuss the key steps for organizing effective home care for your aging parents.

Firstly, it's important to assess the level of care your parents need. This involves a detailed look at their physical abilities, medical conditions, and personal preferences. Understanding the scope of their needs will assist you in determining the type of care necessary, whether it's occasional help with groceries or full-time assistance with daily activities.

Once you've assessed their needs, the next step is to research the types of home care services available. In-home care can range from professional nursing services to non-medical attendant care. There are also specialized providers for conditions such as dementia or physical rehabilitation. Knowing the services that are available allows you to tailor the care to fit your parents' specific requirements.

Creating a care plan is an essential component of organizing home care. A good care plan includes schedules, emergency contacts, medical information, and any other pertinent details that caregivers will need to know. It serves as a roadmap for the care your parents will receive and ensures that everyone involved is on the same page.

Communication is fundamental when coordinating care. Whether you're dealing with siblings, professional caregivers, or your parents themselves, clear and consistent communication helps mitigate misunderstandings and facilitates smoother transitions in care. Frequent family meetings can be an effective way to keep everyone informed and involved.

Funding for home care is another crucial aspect to consider. You'll need to explore all financial options such as long-term care insurance, Medicare, Medicaid, or private pay. It's also beneficial to consult with a financial planner who specializes in elder care to help navigate the complexities of healthcare funding.

Home safety is paramount, and sometimes modifications are necessary to create a safe environment. This can include installing grab bars, ramps, or stairlifts. A professional home assessment can identify potential hazards and suggest appropriate modifications.

When choosing a caregiver or a home care agency, it's essential to conduct thorough interviews, check references, and ensure they are properly licensed and trained. It's important that the caregiver is not only qualified but also a good fit with your parents' personality and needs.

Establishing a routine comes next. Older adults often thrive on routine, and a consistent schedule can aid in reducing anxiety and confusion. Routines also help caregivers provide consistent and efficient care.

It's also necessary to have backup plans in place. Unexpected events, such as a caregiver falling ill or a sudden change in your parent's condition, can happen. Having backup care options and an emergency plan can avert potential crises and provide peace of mind.

Monitoring the quality of care your parents receive is ongoing. Regularly checking in with your parents and their caregivers allows you to stay apprised of their well-being and to make any needed adjustments to the care plan.

Respecting your parents' autonomy and dignity throughout this process cannot be overstated. Involving them in decisions about their care maintains their sense of control and honors their independence.

As your parents' needs evolve, so too must the home care plan. Staying flexible and willing to adjust the plan as circumstances change is a critical element of effective home care.

Keeping detailed records is also part of effective home care management. This includes medical records, care logs, invoices, and contracts. Well-kept records are invaluable, especially when coordinating care with healthcare professionals or dealing with insurance claims.

In times when you or other family members cannot provide the required care, respite care may become necessary. Respite care can provide a much-needed break for family caregivers, while ensuring your parents continue to receive the care they need.

In closing, organizing effective home care is a multifaceted task that requires planning, communication, and accountability. While it can be challenging, the right approach can lead to successful home care that supports your parents' health and happiness. Remember, you're not alone in this journey, and there are numerous resources available to help you provide the best possible care for your aging loved ones.

Chapter 7:
Transitioning to Assisted Living

As we embrace the reality that home care may no longer be the most sustainable option, the thought of transitioning a loved one to assisted living can be wrought with complex emotions and logistical challenges. We've already explored the groundwork required for caregiving, from legal preparations to managing health and at-home care. At this juncture, it's crucial to navigate the delicate process of assessing the most suitable housing options that will provide comfort, expert care, and a sense of community. While daunting, remember that this is a step forward, a move towards ensuring safety, better health supervision, and, perhaps most importantly, companionship for your aging parents. Spearheading this transition involves thorough research, candid family discussions, and a careful balancing act between respecting your parents' independence and acknowledging their care needs. Each family's journey is as unique as the individual at its center; however, the crux of success here lies within a thoughtful, well-informed approach buoyed by empathy, patience, and clear communication.

Evaluating Housing Options

As the journey of caregiving unfolds, the time may come to assess more suitable living situations for your aging parents. Evaluating housing options is a step that demands attention to detail, empathy for your parents' preferences, and a clear understanding of their needs. The process can be overwhelming, but breaking it down into manageable tasks will make it less daunting.

Finding the right assisted living community involves looking at a myriad of factors. The location should be one of the first considerations. Proximity to family members, medical facilities, and the community your parents have grown accustomed to might be important to them. It's not just about convenience; it's about ensuring they feel still connected to their world.

The size and type of facility may greatly impact your parents' comfort and happiness. Some individuals thrive in larger communities offering a wide variety of activities and amenities, while others prefer a smaller, more intimate setting. Listen to your parents' preferences and concerns to guide your search for the right fit.

It's essential to consider the level of care your parents need. Some facilities offer independent living with assistance close at hand, while others provide more intensive nursing and medical care. Understanding the difference between these options and accurately gauging your parents' health will help you select a facility that can adapt to their needs over time.

Site visits are critical in the selection process. These visits allow you and your parents to get a feel for the community culture, interact with staff and residents, and visually inspect the cleanliness and maintenance of the surroundings. Paying attention to how staff members engage with residents can provide insight into the care and attention your parents would receive.

Cost is often a determining factor in choosing an assisted living facility. Transparent pricing structures are crucial. Look for hidden fees, and make sure to understand what is included in the monthly cost. Assess your parents' budget, and consider how long-term care insurance, veterans' benefits, or other resources might help cover expenses.

Ask about staffing ratios and turnover rates. Consistent, well-staffed care is a marker of a quality facility. High turnover can disrupt continuity of care and may indicate underlying issues with the management or work conditions, which could affect the care residents receive.

The range of services and amenities offered can enhance your parents' quality of life considerably. Inquire about dining options, exercise and wellness programs, and social activities. If your parent has a special interest or hobby, find out how the facility might accommodate these passions.

Dietary considerations must not be overlooked. If your parent has specific dietary needs or preferences, check how the facility accommodates these. Meal times are also a social activity in many communities, so you'll want to ensure that this aspect of daily life is fulfilling both nutritionally and socially for your parent.

In addition to the living space itself, consider the facility's policies that impact daily life. This could include everything from pet policies and visiting hours to how medical emergencies are handled. It's crucial that these policies align with your parents' needs and expectations.

Transportation services can be an important aspect of assisted living, particularly if your parents are used to being independent. If they are still driving, check for parking availability. If not, ask about the transport services for medical appointments, shopping trips, or other outings.

Investigate the facility's accreditation and regulatory compliance. An accredited facility typically undergoes rigorous evaluations to ensure they meet certain standards of care and service. Furthermore, understanding state regulations and how facilities adhere to them can provide peace of mind regarding your parents' safety and well-being.

Talk through the programs in place for health and wellness. A facility with an active approach to maintaining the residents' health through preventive measures, rehabilitation services, and easy access to medical care can be invaluable as your parents age and their needs become more complex.

Lastly, remember to involve your parents in the decision-making process as much as possible. After all, it's their home and their life that is changing. Some parents may resist the idea of moving to assisted living, so it's important to show them that their opinions and preferences matter and that you're working together to find the best solution.

The search for the right assisted living facility is a journey filled with many considerations, but it's a necessary step in ensuring your parents' safety, happiness, and health. Take your time, involve your parents, and you will find the place that feels like the right home for this next stage of their lives.

The Move: Preparation and Adjustment

As you approach the significant transition of moving a parent to assisted living, preparation is crucial to a smooth adjustment for everyone involved. The move can be a complex process, blending logistical concerns with deep emotional undercurrents. It's a mixture that requires both practical planning and sensitivity to the emotional needs of your parent.

Finding the right assisted living community is the first step, but what follows is just as critical: preparing for the actual move. This involves downsizing personal belongings, which can be a sensitive subject. It's crucial to approach this task with patience and understanding. Acknowledging the emotional attachment to possessions can make the process less distressing for your parent.

For the move, enlisting the help of professionals or organizing a family workday can alleviate physical and emotional stress. Involving your parent in decisions about what to take can give them a sense of control and respect their autonomy. Remember, the familiar items can greatly contribute to the feeling of homeliness in their new space.

Before the move, discuss the logistics with the assisted living staff to understand move-in day procedures and how to best settle your parent into their new environment. Often, these communities have protocols in place to help new residents acclimate, so tapping into these resources can be beneficial.

Adjustment to assisted living will take time. Initially, your parent might experience a mix of emotions, from relief to sadness or confusion. Staying present during this transition period is essential. Visit often, encourage participation in social activities and maintain open lines of communication with both your parent and the staff.

Conversations with caregivers and fellow residents can provide insight into your parent's adjustment process. These discussions are also valuable opportunities to address any concerns and forge alliances that can offer support and friendship to your parent.

One practical task that can sometimes be overlooked is the customization of your parent's new living space. Personalizing their room with cherished items like photographs, a favorite quilt, or a beloved piece of art can make a world of difference in making them feel at home. It's these personal touches that help bridge the transition from the old environment to the new.

Embracing the community's social environment is also a significant part of the adjustment. Encourage your parent to become involved in activities and social events, which can help foster new friendships and a sense of belonging. This may require some gentle nudging, as the unfamiliarity of new faces and routines can be daunting at first.

Amidst all this change, it's critical to monitor your parent's mental health. Keep an eye out for signs of depression or anxiety, and don't hesitate to seek professional help if needed. The emotional weight of leaving a previous home and starting over cannot be underestimated.

Your involvement in care meetings can be instrumental in ensuring that your parent's needs are being met. Staying informed and asserting your parent's preferences helps in tailoring the care they receive to their individual needs and desires.

During visits, try to establish routines that your parent can look forward to. Whether it's a weekly dinner, a game night, or a shared hobby, these consistent engagements provide something for your parent to anticipate and delight in.

It's essential to respect your parent's autonomy during this period of adjustment. They may be in a new living situation with different support structures, but they remain their own person with their own wishes and needs. Listen to their concerns, support their decisions, and validate their feelings.

Remember that adjustment is not just an event, but a process. It will have its ups and downs and take both time and patience. Patience is particularly important – for both you and your parent. Allow space for your parent to settle in at their own pace, without rushing them or dismissing their emotional responses to the change.

Finally, take care of yourself during this transition. Watching a parent adjust to assisted living can be emotionally taxing, and it's important to acknowledge and attend to your feelings. Seek support when needed, and ensure you have outlets for stress relief and self-care to maintain your own well-being.

Throughout this journey, remember that you're not alone. Millions of families embark on this path every year, and there's a wealth of community resources and professional guidance available. By facing both the logistical and emotional challenges of "The Move: Preparation and Adjustment" with intention and care, you'll be providing your parent with the best foundation possible for their new chapter in assisted living.

Chapter 8:
End-of-Life Considerations

As we navigate the delicate terrain of our parents' final chapter, tensions among siblings can run particularly high, sharpened by differing perspectives on care and the allocation of finances. The emotional weight of a parent's decline often exacerbates familial conflicts, leaving adult children at odds when unity is most needed. It's not uncommon for disagreements to surface over the perceived right course of action, whether it's choosing hospice care, managing pain and comfort, or deciding whether to pursue aggressive treatment for terminal illnesses. In these moments, it's crucial to keep communication lines open, perhaps enlisting the help of a mediator or a healthcare professional experienced in end-of-life care discussions. Throughout this chapter, we'll delve into the practicalities and sensitivities of coordinating care among siblings, emphasizing the importance of consensus and the well-being of the parent at the heart of these crucial decisions. We'll explore how to collectively establish priorities, manage resources wisely, and support one another through the shared journey, always maintaining respect for our parent's dignity and personal wishes.

Palliative Care and Hospice

Time brings us to a critical junction in our caregiving journey: the introduction of palliative care and hospice services. Understanding these care options is essential as your parents age, especially when they're faced with life-limiting illnesses or advanced stages of chronic diseases. This section aims to clarify what each type of care entails and how they can support your parents' quality of life in their final days, weeks, or months.

Palliative care is specialized medical care focused on providing relief from the symptoms and stress of a serious illness. The primary goal is to improve the quality of life for both the patient and their family. It's appropriate at any age and at any stage in a serious illness and can be provided alongside curative treatments. For children taking on the role of caregiver for aging parents, introducing palliative care may be a delicate subject but an important option to consider.

Typically, a team of experts, including doctors, nurses, and other specialists, work together to provide an extra layer of support. Palliative care addresses the emotional, physical, and spiritual needs of the patient, which can be profoundly comforting to them and to you as the caregiver. Discussing the possibility of palliative care with your parents and their doctors can be both a sensitive and empowering conversation, ensuring their wishes are heard and respected.

Once considered, what does the transition to palliative care look like? Initially, it involves assessments by healthcare professionals to determine your parents' needs and the creation of a care plan tailored to those needs. This plan can cover pain management, symptom relief, counseling, and social support. Coordinating with healthcare providers to establish this care can alleviate a great deal of stress and uncertainty for everyone involved.

Hospice care, on the other hand, is designed for people who are in the final phase of a terminal illness. It ensures that patients live out their last moments with dignity and without pain. Hospice provides comprehensive comfort care as well as spiritual and emotional support for the patient and their loved ones. It's an approach that affirms life and regards dying as a natural process, one not to be hastened or postponed.

The eligibility for hospice often requires a doctor's certification that the patient has six months or less to live, assuming the disease follows its natural course. When your parent is ready for hospice, you'll notice the approach to care changes from curative to purely comfort-focused. While hospice can be provided at home, it's also available in hospice facilities, hospitals, and nursing homes.

One of the hardest things you might do as an adult child is to initiate the hospice conversation. Yet, it can also be one of the most loving actions, ensuring your parents receive the compassion and dignity they deserve at the end of life. It's vital to discuss hospice before it becomes an immediate need, so you have the opportunity to make well-informed decisions and honor your parents' wishes regarding end-of-life care.

Both palliative and hospice care emphasize the importance of advanced care planning. Discussing and documenting care preferences early on helps to ensure that medical decisions align with your parents' values and desires. It can also prevent unnecessary interventions and ensure that the focus remains on their comfort and quality of life.

A key part of hospice and palliative care is the support provided to you, the caregiver. Facing the impending loss of a parent is a profound emotional challenge. These services offer bereavement counseling, respite care, and assistance with the practical aspects of care, allowing you to cherish the time you have left with your parent rather than feeling overwhelmed by their care needs.

Knowing when it's time to shift towards palliative care or hospice can be difficult. Look for signs such as a significant decline in health, frequent hospitalizations, or a desire to stop receiving treatments that are no longer effective. Remember, these services are about providing comfort and support, not giving up hope or love.

Once you've engaged hospice or palliative care services, take the time to understand each team member's role and how they contribute to your parent's care. Regular meetings or check-ins can help manage expectations and keep communication open between you, your parent, and the care team. A supportive, multidisciplinary approach ensures that all needs are met with sensitivity and expertise.

It's natural to have many questions regarding these care options. Organizations such as the National Hospice and Palliative Care Organization offer resources and information that can guide you through the specifics of care, eligibility, and how to access these services. Hospice and palliative care programs often have staff available to answer your questions and provide tours or detailed explanations of what you and your parent can expect.

Additionally, financial considerations are a part of final life-stage planning. Medicare, Medicaid, and most insurance plans cover hospice care fully or partially. For palliative care, coverage may vary based on your parent's insurance and the treatment they need. Consult with a financial advisor or social worker specializing in elder care to navigate the costs associated with these services, ensuring that finances do not become an obstacle to comfort and care.

Above all, remember you're not alone in this journey. While it may seem daunting to tackle end-of-life care decisions, there are communities and professionals committed to helping you and your parent through this transition. Lean on the support networks, be open with your feelings and uncertainties, and take each step at a time, honoring the life and legacy of your loved parent.

As we wrap up this discussion on palliative care and hospice, it's essential to realize the significance of these services in providing a gentle, dignified conclusion to a life well-lived. By being proactive in planning and engaging with end-of-life care options, you are upholding your loved one's wishes and ensuring they receive the respect and care they deserve in their final chapter.

Grief, Loss, and Closure

Coping with the terminal phase of a loved one's life inevitably brings about profound grief and a sense of loss. Witnessing the decline of a parent, who has been your caregiver for the longest time, is a role reversal many find difficult to navigate. Through acceptance and understanding, though, one can find the path to closure. It's neither straightforward nor easy, but it is an essential part of the journey.

Grief is an individual experience, nuanced by the relationship you had with your parent and the circumstances of their decline and passing. It's natural to feel a gamut of emotions, ranging from sadness and anger to guilt and regret. These feelings may come in waves or hit all at once and can overwhelm your daily life.

One of the first emotions many grapple with is denial. It serves as a protective buffer, taking the edge off the initial shock. Recognizing this response can help you to move through it and come to terms with the reality of the situation.

As time moves on, you might find yourself in the throes of anger. It's a natural response to feeling helpless in the face of mortality. You may find yourself angry at the world, your parent, or even the healthcare system. Understanding that this anger is a part of the grieving process can help you manage it constructively.

Bargaining is yet another stage of grief. It's the 'what if' and 'if only' thoughts that replay in your mind, often as a way to regain control over the uncontrollable. Remember, these are normal reactions to the pain of loss, and acknowledging them can aid in moving forward.

Depression, distinct from clinical depression, can manifest during the mourning period. It may present as deep sadness, withdrawal from activities, or a general sense of heaviness. It's important to seek support when these feelings interfere with your ability to cope.

Eventually, you'll arrive at acceptance, acknowledging the reality of your parent's passing. This is not to say the pain vanishes, but it becomes manageable. You learn to live with your loss, honoring your parent's memory while continuing with your life.

Finding closure involves creating a narrative that makes sense to you. It could be remembering your parent as they were before their illness, celebrating their life, or recounting their contributions to the world. This re-framing can bring peace.

It's also helpful to participate in rituals or hold memorials to honor your loved one's memory. These gatherings can provide an outlet for shared sorrow and a sense of collective solace. Rituals help us process loss and are a profound step towards healing.

An important aspect of closure is acknowledging any unresolved feelings you have towards your parent. This could involve writing letters, sharing stories with others, or seeking therapy. Finding ways to express these emotions is vital for moving on.

Give yourself permission to grieve on your own terms, and in your own time. Do not measure your process against others or against cultural expectations. Your journey through grief is unique to you, and allowing yourself the space you need is critical for healing.

Remember to lean on your support system throughout this time. Friends, family, support groups, and professional counselors can provide comfort and perspective. They can listen when you need to talk and offer silence when you need reflection.

In the midst of grief, it's important to be mindful of your wellness. Grief can take a toll on your physical health, so maintaining a routine, eating nourishing food, and getting adequate rest is essential.

Finally, as you embrace grieving, also embrace living. Engage with the world around you and allow yourself moments of joy and peace. Such moments do not betray the memory of your loved one but affirm the cycle of life that they were part of.

Grief, loss, and finding closure after the passing of a parent is an intensely personal experience. It's full of contradiction – the need to hold on and the necessity to let go. But in this challenging passage, there is also the potential to grow, to cherish memories, and to discover resilience you may not have known you had.

Chapter 9:
The Caregiver's Well-Being

Moving beyond the previous chapters, where we've navigated the practicalities and emotions surrounding your parent's care, it is vital to put a spotlight on your own well-being as a caregiver. Upholding your health, both mentally and physically, isn't a luxury—it's a necessity that benefits not just you, but also the loved one you're tending to. Juggling appointments, medications, and the heavy emotional toll can lead to an overlooked condition known as caregiver burnout. Within this chapter, we'll delve into strategies that empower you to maintain a balanced life. You'll learn how to recognize the early warning signs of burnout and discover practical steps that can be taken to ensure you're not pouring from an empty cup. Cultivating a resilient mindset, carving out time for your interests, and embracing the power of habit and routine can fortify your sense of self while you deliver unwavering support. Also crucial is the exploration of support systems and respite care options which can provide a much-needed pause and alleviate the weight of caregiver responsibilities. Remember, it's not selfish to focus on your well-being; it's essential. Your vitality directly influences the quality of care you provide and the quality of the shared moments that lie ahead with your parents.

Self-Care and Avoiding Burnout

Tending to the needs of aging parents is an act of love and devotion, but it's critically important for caregivers to remember their own well-being in the process. Introducing self-care practices into your routine isn't an indulgence; it is a crucial part of being an effective caregiver. Without it, you're at an increased risk for burnout—a state of emotional, physical, and mental exhaustion caused by excessive and prolonged stress.

Firstly, let's acknowledge that self-care isn't selfish. It is essential. It's easy to feel that every moment should be dedicated to your parent's care, but that's a one-way ticket to exhaustion. Start simple with a few minutes each day that are just for you—whether it's enjoying a morning coffee in silence, a quick stroll around the block, or a few pages of that book gathering dust on your nightstand.

Next, let's talk about recognizing the signs of caregiver burnout. Are you feeling irritable, having trouble sleeping, or experiencing changes in appetite? Maybe you're feeling detached from your loved ones or finding no joy in activities that used to make you happy. These could all be indicators. It's vital to catch these symptoms early and take proactive steps to address them.

Maintaining a healthy balance between caregiving tasks and your personal life is not without its challenges. However, setting boundaries can help. It's okay to say 'no' or to delegate tasks to others. You can't do it all, and spreading the responsibilities among family members or professional caregivers can lift a significant weight from your shoulders.

Nutrition often takes a backseat when you're overwhelmed with caregiving duties. But consider this—your body is akin to a car; it needs quality fuel to run efficiently. Prioritizing a balanced diet will not only improve your health but provide you with the energy needed to care for your parents. Meal prep on less busy days can make healthy choices easier throughout the week.

Physical activity is another cornerstone of self-care. Regular exercise serves as a stress reliever and mood booster. This doesn't mean you need to sign up for marathon training. Instead, integrate movement into your day: park farther from the store, take the stairs, or dance around to your favorite songs. These little changes can make a big difference.

Sleep cannot be overemphasized. When you're well-rested, everything from your mood to your ability to make decisions improves. Aim for seven to nine hours of sleep per night. If caregiving duties interfere, don't hesitate to ask for overnight help or explore potential devices or services that can provide you with peace of mind so you can rest.

Emotional self-care is just as important as physical. Caregiving can be a roller coaster of emotions. Find time for activities that calm your mind and soothe your soul. This could be journaling, meditating, engaging in a hobby, or simply talking to a friend. Don't underestimate the power of a good laugh or a good cry—they're both therapeutic.

Building a support system is another critical aspect of avoiding burnout. Connect with friends, join a support group, or even seek professional counseling. It's important to have a safe space where you can voice your frustrations, concerns, and feelings without fear of judgment.

Consider practicing mindfulness and gratitude exercises. Mindfulness can keep you grounded and help you better cope with the stresses of caregiving by bringing your focus back to the present moment. And, reflecting on things you're grateful for each day can shift your perspective and help reduce stress.

Respite care is a godsend for many caregivers. This temporary relief allows you to take time for yourself, whether it's for a few hours or a few days. Use this time to recharge. Maybe take that weekend getaway you've been daydreaming about or even just a day to yourself to do nothing at all.

Learning to let go of guilt is key to your mental health. You might feel guilty for taking time for yourself or for feeling frustrated and tired. Remember, these feelings are normal and don't reflect your love or commitment to your parents. Self-care does not mean you care any less; it means you understand the need to maintain your health to provide the best care possible.

Finally, embrace flexibility. Your caregiving journey will evolve, and your self-care strategies may need to adjust as well. What works for you now may not work in six months, and that's okay. The crux of avoiding burnout lies in the ability to adapt and address your needs as they change over time.

Remember, caregiving is a significant undertaking, and it's okay to feel overwhelmed at times. If or when that happens, reach out. There are innumerable resources and services available that can help. Looking after your well-being ensures that you'll be better equipped to care for your parents, who rely on your strength and support.

Caring for aging parents requires compassion, patience, and resilience. By prioritizing self-care and being mindful of burnout, you'll not only be taking care of your parents but also honoring your own needs in the process. This balance is not only desirable but necessary for the wellbeing of everyone involved.

Seeking Support and Respite

Caring for aging parents is a profound testament to love and responsibility. Yet, it can also be a source of immense stress and fatigue. It's crucial to recognize that no one is equipped to do it all alone. Seeking support and respite is not just a luxury—it's necessary for the sustainability of your caregiving journey.

An effective strategy for finding support may begin with family meetings to discuss the division of tasks. Understand that not all siblings or family members have equal capacity to contribute, but most can offer support in varied ways. It may be logistical, financial, or emotional, but each contribution eases the burden and provides a network for the caregiver.

Additionally, looking beyond your immediate circle is important. Local support groups can provide a platform for sharing experiences and strategies. In these groups, you may find comfort in knowing others face similar challenges. The camaraderie found here can be a steady source of strength, easing the sense of isolation that sometimes accompanies caregiving.

Professional counseling services should also be considered vital. As emotions ebb and flow, a counselor or therapist can help navigate complex feelings in a safe and constructive environment. They can suggest coping mechanisms and stress-relief strategies specifically tailored to caregivers.

Respite care, too, is a key component of a support system. This can be anything from enlisting the help of home care services for a few hours a week, to arranging short-term stays at assisted living facilities. Respite gives you a necessary pause to recharge and attend to your own needs.

Technology has opened up new avenues for support as well. Online communities can be accessed at any time, providing a 24/7 lifeline to others who understand your situation. Mobile health monitoring tools can ease worries about leaving your parent unattended, which can free you up to take breaks with peace of mind.

Volunteering services in your community may offer unexpected sources of aid. Sometimes local civic organizations, religious groups, or nonprofits have programs designed to assist caregivers. These can range from driving your parent to appointments, to delivering meals, or even providing companionship.

Educational workshops and seminars can not only offer new caregiving skills but also introduce you to a network of like-minded individuals. Learning more about the conditions your parent may be facing will empower you with knowledge and potentially new contacts who can offer practical advice.

Options for professional respite care can also be researched through your local Area Agency on Aging. They can guide you to vetted services and financial assistance programs for respite care. By tapping into these resources, you're not only finding help, you're ensuring the help is reliable and tailored to the elder population.

Taking care of yourself is not a separate task from caregiving—it's a part of it. This includes physical exercise, which can help manage stress and keep you healthy. Never underestimate the power of a quick walk or workout in lifting your mood and giving you an energy boost.

Maintaining a hobby or personal interest is also vital. It's tempting to put your own life on hold, but remaining engaged in your passions can be rejuvenating and prevents resentment from taking root.

Time management skills can greatly increase the efficiency of your caregiving duties. By organizing your day and delegating non-essential tasks, you'll find pockets of time for yourself. This might be a few moments of meditation, a calming bath, or simply reading a book.

Seeking support is not an admission of failure but an acknowledgment of your limits. Being proactive about arranging for time away from your caregiving responsibilities can help maintain your wellbeing, and in turn, improve the quality of care you can provide for your parent.

Lastly, never hesitate to reach out to your healthcare provider if you find the stress overwhelming. They can do regular check-ups not just for your parent, but for you as well, ensuring that you're not neglecting your own health needs.

Remember, in order to take care of someone else, you must first take care of yourself. Seeking support and respite is not a luxury—it's an essential part of the caregiving process that helps you sustain the marathon that is caregiving, with love and resilience.

Chapter 10:
Staying Connected and Engaged

In the continuum of caregiving, maintaining the bond between you and your aging parents is a cornerstone that supports not just their well-being, but your own. As we transition from discussing the caregiver's health in the previous chapter, it's vital to emphasize the importance of nurturing relationships and facilitating enriching social interactions for our loved ones. Creating opportunities for your parents to stay involved with family, friends, and their community can counter feelings of isolation and help preserve their identity and sense of purpose. It's equally important to embrace technology's role in bridging distances—using video calls, social media, and other digital platforms can keep your parents feeling present and connected. But staying engaged isn't solely about social connections; it involves integrating activities that spark joy and stimulation, whether through hobbies, cultural experiences, or simple shared moments with you. In this chapter, we'll explore methods to weave this tapestry of connection—keeping the golden threads of your parents' personalities shining through as they age.

Fostering Relationships with Aging Parents

As our parents age, the fabric of our family dynamics can shift dramatically. This phase of life brings an opportunity to deepen our relationships with our parents, understanding their needs while respecting their independence and dignity. Fostering these relationships requires empathy, patience, and an emphasis on maintaining connections that enrich everyone involved.

Maintaining a strong relationship with aging parents isn't just about offering care; it's about preserving the emotional bonds that have been built over a lifetime. It's common to confront a mix of emotions as you take on more responsibilities in your parents' lives, but it's also a time to rediscover each other in new and meaningful ways.

Communication is the key to a healthy relationship. Keep conversations regular and open. Be interested in your parents' views, stories, and daily experiences. Encourage them to share their thoughts and feelings, and actively listen. It's important for them to feel heard and understood, not just looked after.

While respecting their independence, it's beneficial to participate in activities together. This might mean sharing a hobby, going for walks, attending community events, or simply enjoying a meal together. Shared experiences can boost their morale and reinforce the familial bond.

Revisiting cherished memories can brighten your parents' spirits. Go through old photo albums, tell stories, and share laughs about past family adventures. This can be particularly comforting and a strong reminder of the beautiful moments you've shared throughout the years.

It's vital to respect your parents' autonomy. As much as you may want to protect or help them with everything, allowing them the space to make decisions, where they're able to, fosters independence and self-respect. Balance is crucial; being too protective can sometimes feel patronizing or oppressive.

Physical touch can be an essential element of connection, especially if your parents are open to it. A hug, a pat on the back, or simply holding their hand can communicate love and care beyond words, providing comfort and reassurance during a stage of life that can often feel isolating.

Remember the importance of laughter. Humor can be a wonderful tonic in lightening the mood and connecting with each other. Share jokes, funny stories, or watch a comedy together. It's a natural way to bond and cope with the stresses that can accompany aging and caregiving.

Be attentive to your parents' changing needs, but don't lose sight of who they are beyond their age or health issues. Honor their life stories, recognize their accomplishments, and acknowledge their value and place in the world. This respect for their personhood is critical to a thriving relationship.

Although your role may involve more responsibilities now, don't let the caregiver duties entirely overshadow the parent-child relationship. Keep the lines of communication as bilateral as possible. Encourage your parents to still be there for you in ways they can, whether that's giving advice, listening, or sharing in your life's events.

It's important to acknowledge that some days will be tough. Patience will sometimes wear thin, and frustrations may surface. In those moments, remember the love at the core of the relationship. Take a step back, breathe, and approach situations with compassion for yourself and your parents.

Don't hesitate to include your parents in decision-making that affects them, whenever it's practical. Whether it's about their health, living arrangements, or daily routines, making decisions together strengthens trust and ensures that their voices are always part of the conversation.

As your parents age, fostering a relationship also means being their advocate. When interfacing with healthcare professionals or handling bureaucratic tasks, keep your parents' preferences and best interests in mind. These efforts demonstrate your commitment to their well-being and your respect for their life choices.

Lastly, don't forget to enlist the support of other family members, friends, and professional services when necessary. A collaborative approach not only eases the burden on you but also adds a rich tapestry of care and interaction for your parents, ensuring they are surrounded by a loving and engaged community.

Fostering the relationship with your aging parents is a delicate dance of support, respect, engagement, and love. It's about creating new memories while cherishing the old ones, and navigating the complexities of life's later chapters together. By maintaining these connections, you honor the relationship's history and build a foundation for the journey ahead.

Incorporating Social Activities and Technology

Caring for aging parents introduces a complex blend of responsibilities, emotions, and logistics. Among the pivotal elements to promote a fulfilling quality of life for our parents is ensuring continued social interaction and embracing the benefits of technology. This section delves into practical strategies to integrate both social activities and technology into the lives of our aging loved ones, contributing to their well-being and sense of connectedness.

It's crucial to understand that social activity is not merely an option, but a necessity for the emotional and cognitive health of older adults. Social interactions can stave off loneliness and depression, which are common challenges as one ages. Therefore, it's important to encourage regular engagement with friends, family, and community. This might take the form of weekly card games, book clubs, or simply sharing meals with others.

Meanwhile, technology can be a double-edged sword. On one hand, it holds immense potential to connect and enrich the lives of seniors. On the other, it can be daunting for those who weren't raised in the digital era. Approach this disparity with patience and empathy. Introducing simple-to-use devices, such as tablets with intuitive touch screens, can be a great starting point. Prioritize setting up video calls with family members, which can be a tangible lifeline for parents who live alone or are at a distance from their loved ones.

One cannot reinforce enough the value of including your parents in the decision-making process regarding social activities. It's important to listen to their preferences and comfort levels. Some may relish the opportunity to attend a dance class or a lecture series, while others may prefer more intimate gatherings or one-on-one visits.

When integrating technology, think about the services that could enhance your parent's life. For instance, meal delivery apps can bring diverse dining experiences into their home. Online classes offer avenues for continuous learning and hobbies. Offering to set up and walk them through the use of these services can ease them into a more connected lifestyle.

Moreover, there's potential in social media for keeping your parents engaged. Platforms like Facebook can enable them to keep up with family and reconnect with long-lost friends. However, it's critical to educate them on privacy settings and digital security to keep their online experience safe.

For seniors who show resistance to technology, start with the basics. Teach them to send and receive text messages or emails. This small step opens a valuable channel for daily communication and provides a sense of achievement that can motivate further learning.

Keep in mind the accessibility features present in many devices. They can make a world of difference for parents with visual or hearing impairments. Features like text-to-speech, large font sizes, and high-contrast settings can transform frustrating attempts into successful interactions with technology.

Don't forget to celebrate the wins, no matter how small. When your parent learns to take a selfie, share it with pride in the family group chat. These moments of joy can encourage them to continue exploring what technology has to offer.

It's also worth investigating local senior centers or community groups that offer technology workshops specifically designed for older adults. These programs can provide a more structured environment for learning and help them to build confidence in their abilities.

Loneliness can be more than a feeling; it can lead to significant health issues. Organizing virtual family reunions via video conferencing platforms can simulate the warmth of being together and remind your parents that they are an integral part of a loving circle.

Similarly, incorporating smart home technology can contribute to a safer living environment while promoting independence. Features such as voice-activated assistants, automated lighting, and medical alert systems add layers of support that can provide peace of mind to both you and your parents.

On the other hand, also take time to facilitate in-person gatherings—taking into account mobility and transportation needs. Perhaps establishing a carpool roster among family and friends can help in getting your parent to social events and appointments.

Finally, it's paramount to remind ourselves that teaching and learning are reciprocal. While we might be introducing our parents to the digital world, they share with us the intangible wisdom of their years. Celebrating this exchange enriches the caregiver-parent relationship and paves the way for a richer understanding and appreciation of each other's worlds.

By integrating thoughtfully chosen social activities and user-friendly technology into the lives of our aging parents, we widen their world. We enable them to maintain a sense of community and belonging, which is essential for their overall happiness and health. With each shared video call, online game, or new tech skill acquired, we are reinforcing that even as they age, our parents remain connected and valued members of the family tapestry.

Chapter 11:
Navigating Memory Care

When your parent's memory begins to fade, the path forward can be daunting and filled with nuanced challenges that test both your patience and emotional fortitude. Entering the world of memory care means understanding the intricate stages of dementia and Alzheimer's disease, learning to communicate effectively despite the impairments, and finding comfort in the daily routines that provide your loved ones with a sense of normalcy and security. Memory care requires a delicate balance of honoring who your parents have been while also adapting to the reality of their cognitive changes. It's a process that can be incredibly trying, but it's not one you have to face alone. This chapter serves as a foundation for the uncharted territory of dementia care, guiding you towards specialized memory care options and introducing therapies that respect the dignity of your loved ones while addressing the intricacies of their condition. With every turn of the page, you'll find strategies to navigate this complex landscape with empathy, advocating for your parents' needs, and ultimately, ensuring they receive the best care possible amidst the ebbs and flows of memory loss.

Understanding Dementia and Alzheimer's Disease

When it comes to caring for aging parents, understanding their particular health challenges is crucial. Dementia and Alzheimer's disease are progressive conditions that impact memory, cognitive function, and the ability to perform everyday tasks. As we delve into this important topic, it's essential to differentiate these terms. Dementia is the overarching term that describes a range of symptoms associated with a decline in mental function severe enough to interfere with daily life. Alzheimer's disease, on the other hand, is the most common type of dementia, accounting for an estimated 60 to 80 percent of cases.

Recognizing the early signs of dementia can be challenging. Initial symptoms often include short-term memory loss, difficulty finding the right words, trouble understanding visual images and spatial relationships, and impaired judgment or decision-making. These signs are frequently subtle and can easily be mistaken for normal aging or stress. However, as the disease progresses, symptoms become more pronounced, affecting the individual's ability to communicate, reason, and recognize familiar faces and environments.

Alzheimer's disease follows a particular pattern of progression, generally characterized in stages. It's vital to note that while the stages provide a framework, each person's journey can vary. In the early stage, known as mild Alzheimer's, individuals may still function independently but might be experiencing memory lapses. As the disease progresses to the moderate stage, more intensive assistance with daily activities becomes necessary. In the final stage, severe Alzheimer's, communication becomes limited, and physical functions significantly decline.

Caring for a parent with dementia or Alzheimer's disease requires not only practical adjustments but also a deep well of patience and understanding. Changes in behavior and personality, such as mood swings, agitation, and even aggression, can be distressing for both the individual and their caregivers. It's important to remember that these behaviors are manifestations of the disease and not intentional.

To effectively navigate memory care for a loved one, it's crucial to educate oneself about the disease process. Familiarizing yourself with the expected progression helps in planning for care needs as they change. This knowledge base allows you to approach caregiving with a level of foresight, preparing for new challenges before they arise.

Securing an accurate diagnosis is a foundational step in the journey. A variety of tests and evaluations, often involving a neurologist or geriatrician, can help determine if your parent's symptoms result from Alzheimer's disease or another form of dementia. This process can also rule out reversible causes of cognitive impairment, such as vitamin deficiencies or medication effects. An early diagnosis opens the door to treatment options that may offer some symptom relief and allows for more time to plan for the future.

While there is no cure for Alzheimer's disease, certain medications can help manage symptoms. These treatments aim to maintain cognitive function for as long as possible and to combat the behavioral issues that often accompany memory decline. It's also beneficial to explore complementary therapies that can enhance quality of life, such as music therapy, art therapy, and physical activity tailored to your parent's abilities.

Communication techniques are an essential part of dementia care. It's important to create a positive environment that reduces confusion and agitation. Simple adjustments, such as reducing background noise, speaking slowly, and using straightforward sentences, can dramatically improve interactions with your parent. Nonverbal cues are also significant; maintaining eye contact and offering reassuring touch can convey love and support even when words fail.

Another aspect of caring for a parent with these conditions is creating a safe and supportive home environment. Modifications might be necessary to prevent falls, wandering, and other safety risks. Additionally, establishing routines can provide a sense of stability for someone with dementia, who may feel overwhelmed by a constantly changing environment.

As we navigate these complexities, it's essential to acknowledge the emotional toll it can take on you, the caregiver. It's not uncommon to experience feelings of loss, grief, and frustration as you watch your parent's personality and abilities diminish. Ensuring you also have access to support through caregiver groups or counseling can make a significant difference in your ability to provide sustained care.

When home-based care becomes too challenging, or when the progression of the disease necessitates a more specialized setting, considering a memory care facility may be the next step. These facilities are designed to provide a secure environment with structured activities and programs that address the needs of individuals with memory impairment. Staff in these settings are specially trained to manage the unique challenges of dementia care.

In conclusion, understanding dementia and Alzheimer's disease serves as the groundwork for providing compassionate and effective care. It's about staying informed, anticipating changes, and adapting to meet your parent's evolving needs. As we move forward, we'll explore specialized memory care options and therapies that can further aid in this journey, supporting both those who suffer from memory conditions and their caregivers.

Finally, it's important to remember that navigating this path involves an ever-changing landscape. You may face difficult decisions, unexpected developments, and new demands on your resilience and resources. Being well-informed and prepared can't prevent all the difficulties, but it can help mitigate them, ensuring that your parent's dignity and well-being are maintained as much as possible throughout this journey.

Whether you're at the beginning stages of recognizing your parent's memory issues or deeper into the management of their care, remember that you're not alone. There are resources and communities available to support you. Together, we can provide our loved ones with the care and affection they deserve in these later chapters of their lives.

Specialized Memory Care and Therapies

As we journey deeper into the realm of memory care, it's essential to understand that dementia and Alzheimer's disease are more than just medical conditions; they have the capacity to transform everything familiar to our loved ones. Specialized memory care, which encompasses a range of therapies and interventions, is designed specifically to address the unique needs of individuals with these diagnoses. Embarking on this path can often feel overwhelming, but knowing your options is the first step toward providing the best care possible.

Memory care units, often found within assisted living facilities or nursing homes, offer structured environments optimized to reduce confusion and agitation for residents with cognitive impairments. These dedicated spaces are equipped with enhanced security measures to prevent wandering—a common and potentially dangerous symptom of dementia-related illnesses. Within these secure walls, residents receive personalized care tailored to their specific stage of memory loss.

When exploring memory care options, look for facilities that offer comprehensive programs which marry traditional health care with innovative therapies aimed at maintaining or improving cognitive function. You'll want to find a place that feels more like a community than an institution, where your loved one will be treated with dignity and respect. The staff should not only have specialized training in dementia care but also exhibit patience, empathy, and a deep understanding of the complexities associated with the disease.

Therapeutic interventions play a pivotal role in specialized memory care and can include a variety of approaches. One such approach is cognitive therapy, where individuals engage in tasks and activities designed to stimulate the brain. These may involve problem-solving exercises, memory games, or other cognitive challenges that can help slow the progression of symptoms and retain mental functions longer.

On the other hand, sensory therapies leverage a person's senses to evoke positive emotions and memories. Music therapy, for example, can help unlock memories and enable moments of connection even as verbal communication becomes challenging. Similarly, art therapy encourages expression through creative activities, sometimes reigniting sparks of personality and individuality that seemed lost.

Physical activity is another cornerstone of memory care. Exercise programs designed for the elderly, including those with cognitive impairments, can improve overall health and help maintain motor skills. Even something as seemingly simple as walking or seated exercises can make a significant difference in your parent's well-being.

Don't overlook the impact of a consistent routine, either. Routine can be grounding for those with memory impairments, providing a structure that helps to orient and reduce anxiety. Specialized memory care programs should emphasize regular schedules, including set times for meals, activities, and resting, to establish a sense of stability and security.

Social interaction is yet another critical aspect of specialized memory care. Social therapies aim to keep individuals connected to others, facilitating group activities that foster a sense of belonging and help maintain communication skills. When selecting a memory care facility, observe the interactions between residents and note the different types of group sessions available.

It's also worth noting that specialized memory care often includes end-of-life care. This can involve palliative care approaches that prioritize comfort and quality of life, even as your loved one's memory continues to fade. These services are provided with compassion, ensuring that the individual's final days are spent with dignity.

Nutritional care should also be a factor in your decision-making process. Cognitive impairments can sometimes lead to changes in diet or eating habits, and memory care facilities are typically adept at handling these challenges. They can provide meals tailored to dietary needs and preferences, ensuring your parent receives proper nutrition, which can, in turn, impact overall health and cognitive function.

In addition to these therapeutic approaches, many memory care facilities are incorporating cutting-edge technologies and programs into their care regimens. Virtual reality, for instance, is being used to take residents on virtual tours of places they may remember from their past, providing comfort and stimulation. Look for a facility that keeps abreast of such advancements and thoughtfully integrates them into their care practices.

When evaluating specialized memory care programs, take note of the facility's approach to individualized care plans. The understanding that each person's journey with dementia is unique is fundamental to providing effective care. These tailored plans take into account the individual's history, preferences, and current abilities, and are regularly updated as needs evolve.

Throughout all these therapies and care approaches, communication with family members should be a priority for the memory care team. Regular updates and involvement in care planning can ensure that you, as a caregiver, are informed and can collaborate with the care team to provide the best support for your loved one.

Lastly, while the focus is often on the individual receiving care, consider the support the facility offers to family members. Effective memory care facilities often provide counseling, support groups, and educational sessions to help families cope with the challenges of caring for a loved one with dementia. These resources are invaluable as you navigate this difficult journey alongside your parent.

In summary, specialized memory care and therapies are about creating an environment that is safe, nurturing, and dignified, with a multipronged approach that includes mental stimulation, physical activity, sensory experiences, social engagement, and personal care. It's about honoring the person behind the condition, connecting with them in the present, and ensuring their comfort each step of the way. As caregivers, our primary focus is to help our aging parents live out their days with the best quality of life possible, surrounded by care that not only understands dementia but respects the individual it affects.

Chapter 12:
Advocating for Your Parent

Stepping into the role of advocate for your aging parent means becoming their voice in situations where they might be unheard or misunderstood. As their staunchest ally, you'll ensure their needs are met with the respect and dignity they deserve. Whether you're communicating with doctors, coordinating with insurance companies, or making decisions about their care, it's crucial to be informed, assertive, and empathetic. You'll navigate complex medical jargon, stand firm against bureaucratic red tape, and, at times, make difficult choices. By arming yourself with knowledge and a deep understanding of your parent's wishes and rights, you'll be their pillar of support through the intricacies of the healthcare system. Remember, advocating doesn't just mean speaking for them—it means listening to them, honoring their autonomy, and empowering them to make their own choices whenever possible. In this chapter, we'll explore the subtle art of advocacy that balances speaking out with stepping back, ensuring your parent's voice is amplified, not overshadowed.

Interacting with Healthcare Professionals

When advocating for your aging parent, it's crucial to develop effective communication with healthcare professionals. Understand they are your allies in ensuring your parent receives the best care possible, but also remember that you're an essential part of your parent's healthcare team. An open line of communication can make a significant difference in the treatment and well-being of your loved one.

The first step is to be prepared for medical appointments. You'll want to gather any relevant information such as medical history, medications, and recent changes in health or behavior. Take notes during appointments and ask for clarifications if needed. Your role is to provide context for your parent's health situation that they might not remember or feel comfortable sharing.

Don't hesitate to ask questions. Healthcare professionals appreciate when family members are engaged and informed. This might include asking about the purpose of medications, alternative treatments, or implications of potential side effects. A thorough understanding will allow you to better oversee your parent's care plan.

It's also important to respect the expertise of the professionals while standing firm in your advocacy role. If something doesn't sit right with you or clashes with your knowledge about your parent's preferences or history, speak up. Your input is vital in creating a care plan that's in your parent's best interest.

Among the most challenging scenarios are complex medical discussions. In such situations, it can help to have another family member or a close friend accompany you to lend support and serve as an additional listener. Two sets of ears are better than one, particularly when dealing with intricate health details or difficult decisions.

Building a relationship with your parent's primary care physician is particularly important, as they often coordinate other specialist treatments and therapies. Make an effort to meet the physician, express your willingness to collaborate, and share any concerns you may have. A good rapport with the primary physician can ensure more holistic care for your parent.

Remember the importance of privacy and confidentiality. While advocating for your parent, always ensure that you have the appropriate permissions to discuss their health information with professionals. This usually requires a HIPAA authorization form, which your parent would need to sign while they are competent to give consent.

Clear communication also extends to the comprehension of potential procedures or hospitalizations. Should such scenarios arise, ensure you understand the goals, benefits, and risks associated with any proposed interventions. Your role includes helping your parent understand these as well, should they be able to participate in the decision-making.

Additionally, when dealing with healthcare professionals, don't neglect the human element. Nurses, doctors, and support staff are more likely to go above and beyond for patients they see are cared for and respected by their families. A kind word and acknowledgement of their efforts can foster a more positive atmosphere for everyone involved.

Technology can also be an asset in your interactions. Many healthcare providers now offer patient portals that can be incredibly helpful. These portals often allow you to ask questions, set appointments, request prescription refills, and even view test results online. Being tech-savvy can streamline the care process considerably.

When your parent is hospitalized or in a care facility, don't shy away from participating in discharge planning. This critical phase involves understanding post-discharge instructions, coordination of follow-up care, and managing transitions to other care settings or home. You must be proactive during this stage to avoid any potential complications.

Should conflicts arise with the healthcare team, it's key to remain diplomatic and solution-focused. While it's important to be assertive on behalf of your parent, maintaining a respectful tone and seeking mutual understanding can prevent unnecessary antagonism and lead to better outcomes.

In cases of chronic illness or when facing end-of-life decisions, consider seeking out a case manager or patient advocate. These professionals specialize in navigating complex healthcare systems and can offer invaluable assistance in coordinating care and communicating with multiple healthcare providers.

Finally, make sure to keep accurate records of all healthcare interactions, including names, dates, and the substance of conversations. These records can be crucial in tracking your parent's care journey and are especially important should you need to refer back to specific discussions or decisions that were made.

Advocating for your parent in the healthcare realm is no small feat. It requires patience, persistence, and a willingness to learn and adapt. By effectively interacting with healthcare professionals, you'll ensure your parent receives the best possible care and that their wishes are respected throughout their healthcare journey.

Navigating the Healthcare System

When it comes to advocating for your aging parents, understanding how to navigate the healthcare system becomes a central part of your role. You'll find that it can be labyrinthine, but with the right approach, you can effectively guide your parents through it. In this section, we'll explore strategies for doing just that.

First, it's important to have all pertinent medical information and records organized. This includes understanding their current health plans, medication lists, former surgeries or hospitalizations, and any ongoing treatments. Maintaining an up-to-date health summary can prevent unnecessary repeat tests and assist new healthcare providers in delivering coordinated care.

Heath insurance is another critical aspect of the healthcare maze. It's imperative that you have a deep understanding of your parents' insurance coverage. This means knowing the ins and outs of their Medicare, Medicaid, or private insurance plans. What is covered? What isn't? Who are the in-network providers? Such questions are foundational in making informed decisions on behalf of your parents.

Healthcare institutions often have patient advocates or care coordinators on staff. Familiarize yourself with these roles as they can be vital in assisting you to navigate through various health services. They are there to help manage care, explain complex medical terms, and support decision-making when your parent is facing multiple healthcare options.

Primary care physicians (PCPs) are usually the quarterbacks of any healthcare team. They should be your first point of contact for non-emergency medical issues. Building a strong relationship with your parent's PCP allows for better continuity of care and assists in reducing hospital visits, which can be unsettling and exhausting for older adults.

When specialists are involved, coordination becomes key. Keep a list of all medical professionals providing care, along with their contact information. Ensure that communication channels are open between your parent's healthcare providers to facilitate a united front in managing health issues.

Prepare for appointments by making a list of questions and concerns. Accompanying your parent, if possible, can help to ensure that all their needs are addressed and their questions answered. Taking notes during the visit can also be immensely helpful in retaining important information discussed.

Decoding medical bills and insurance statements can be overwhelming. If discrepancies or questions arise, don't hesitate to reach out to the billing departments of healthcare providers or the insurance company itself. Keeping a log of these communications can aid in resolving disputes that may occur.

As we age, the risk of emergency health situations increases. Familiarizing yourself with the emergency protocols and services in your parents' area can save valuable time and reduce stress in a crisis. Know the location of the closest hospital, and understand when and how to use services like ambulances.

For chronic conditions or serious health issues, consider seeking out a professional case manager or a geriatric care manager. These professionals can offer specialized insights and help develop a long-term care plan that's tailored to your parent's individual needs.

Utilizing technology can enhance the caregiving process within the healthcare system. Electronic health records, online patient portals, and telemedicine services provide convenience and accessibility. They can enable you to schedule appointments, renew prescriptions, and even attend virtual consultations with physicians.

To be prepared for potential hospitalizations, have a hospital bag ready with essentials such as clothing, toiletries, and a copy of key medical documents. Knowing the patient's rights and the hospital's protocols can also lead to improved patient care and family involvement.

After a hospital stay, discharge planning is a critical phase. Ensure that you understand the aftercare instructions and any prescribed medications. Arrange follow-up visits and be aware of signs that might indicate a need for readmission.

It's also beneficial to be aware of patient support programs and community resources that can aid in recovery, such as rehabilitation services, support groups, or transportation services. These can greatly ease the burden of aftercare for both your parent and you.

Lastly, try to stay informed about changes in healthcare policies and insurance benefits that could affect your parents' care. This may include keeping abreast with updates on Medicare, new healthcare legislation, or changes in coverage provided by their insurance.

Understand that navigating the healthcare system is a dynamic process that requires patience, attention to detail, and a proactive approach. As you advocate for your parent, you'll become more adept at managing the complexities and will be better prepared to support their well-being and dignity throughout the healthcare journey.

Chapter 13:
The Continuum of Care

Caring for an aging parent is a journey that evolves and unfolds in stages, with each phase carrying its own set of challenges and rewards. It's about finding a delicate balance between support and independence, health management, and emotional well-being. This continuum of care is not a fixed path, but rather a fluid progression that requires adaptability, patience, and an open heart. As we've journeyed through the previous chapters, we've explored everything from the initial signs that care is needed to the compassionate handling of end-of-life considerations. Although this chapter marks the conclusion of the book, it's important to remember that your journey with your parent will continue to evolve, with each day presenting a new opportunity to strengthen the bonds of love and care.

The provision of care is inherently dynamic, and it often involves navigating complex healthcare systems, addressing legal and financial concerns, and, significantly, managing the emotional landscape that comes with role reversal. Amidst all these responsibilities, don't lose sight of the fact that the care you give exists on a spectrum that ebb and flows with the needs and health of your parent. It requires you to be as forgiving and gentle with yourself as you are with them. Recognize your limitations and remember it's crucial to reach out for help when you need it. Engaging with caregiving support groups, seeking respite when necessary, and utilizing available resources can provide you with the strength needed to continue in your role.

Finally, beneath the logistical tasks and daily routines lies the true essence of caregiving—a profound expression of love. Embrace the joys that come from the little moments: a shared laugh, an old story retold, or a quiet afternoon spent together. These instances are the threads that weave the tapestry of your continuum of care into something truly invaluable. As each day passes, hold onto the knowledge that the time and care you dedicate to your aging parents is an irreplaceable gift to them, and to yourself. Whatever the future holds, your journey together is enriched by every act of kindness, every decision made in love, and every memory cherished along the way.

Appendix A:
Resource Directory

As we embrace the role of caregivers, it's crucial to know that we are not alone on this journey. There are a plethora of resources at our disposal that can offer assistance, guidance, and support. This directory is a simple-to-navigate compendium tailored to help you find state and federal resources alongside online and community support options, so you and your aging parents can access the help you need when you need it.

State and Federal Resources

The landscape of state and federal resources is wide-ranging, designed to assist seniors and their caregivers in various ways. Each state provides unique programs and services, which often complement federal offerings to support aging adults.

- *Area Agencies on Aging (AAA):* These local agencies can be invaluable, providing information on services such as meal programs, transportation, and caregiver support groups in your area. Locate your nearest AAA by searching the Eldercare Locator at **https://eldercare.acl.gov/**.

- *Medicare:* For comprehensive information on Medicare parts A, B, C, and D, as well as coverage specifics for aging individuals, visit **https://www.medicare.gov/**. Additionally, they have resources for caregivers to help understand billing, rights, and what's covered.

- *Social Security Administration:* To understand the retirement, disability, Social Security, and Medicare benefits your parents might be entitled to, peruse **https://www.ssa.gov/**.

- *Veterans Affairs:* If your parent is a veteran, they may be eligible for additional health care, financial assistance, and housing benefits. Check **https://www.va.gov/** to learn more about the specific qualifications and services available.

- *BenefitsCheckUp®:* Operated by the National Council on Aging, this service can help you find state and federal assistance programs for seniors, from help with medications to utility costs. Visit **https://www.benefitscheckup.org/** to conduct a free and confidential search.

Online and Community Support

In addition to state and federal programs, a rich tapestry of online and community support exists to help you along the caregiving path.

- *Family Caregiver Alliance:* This national center offers advice, advocacy, and support services to those caring for a relative with chronic or health-related needs. Their website **https://www.caregiver.org/** offers a wealth of information.

- *Alzheimer's Association:* For families navigating memory care, the Alzheimer's Association provides resources, support groups, and a 24/7 helpline at **https://www.alz.org/**.

- *Caregiver Action Network:* This network furnishes caregivers with tips, toolkits, and peer forums to share experiences and wisdom. Access their resources at **https://www.caregiveraction.org/**.

- *Next Avenue:* A digital platform that offers thoughtful stories and information on aging and caregiving topics can be found at **https://www.nextavenue.org/**.

- *Meetup Groups:* Local Meetup groups can connect you with fellow caregivers in your area for mutual support and sharing of best practices. Visit **https://www.meetup.com/** and search for caregiver groups in your community.

Empower yourself as a caregiver by harnessing these resources. Whether it's gaining insights on legal matters, finding emotional support, or understanding intricate healthcare nuances, these tools can offer substantial help. You're making a difference in your parents' lives, and it's essential to remember that an entire network is ready to support you on this path.

With this Resource Directory, may you find both the strength to carry on and the knowledge that a collective support system surrounds you and your loved ones. These resources serve as a compass and a companion through the chapters of your caregiving story.

State and Federal Resources When stepping into the pivotal role of caring for an aging parent, knowing your state and federal resource options is crucial for providing the best care and support. These resources can offer financial assistance, medical care, supportive services, and information to aid your caregiving journey.

State resources can vary significantly, depending on where you live. Most states have an Aging Services Division that provides programs and services tailored to the older population. It may include adult day care, meal services, transportation, or respite care to give you a well-deserved break. To find out about the specific programs available in your state, you'll need to connect with your local Area Agency on Aging. They will be your gateway to understanding the full range of services and benefits available to you and your parent.

Similarly, federal resources offer a wide range of programs that can provide financial assistance and support. Medicare, the federally funded healthcare program for those over 65, covers many medical expenses such as hospital stays and doctor visits. Understanding what Medicare covers is essential because it dictates which medical and health-related costs you or your parent will be responsible for. There's also Medicaid, which is an assistance program for those with limited income and assets. While Medicaid is federal, it is state-administered, and eligibility can vary, so it's important to check your state's specific requirements.

Social Security also plays a key role in providing financial support for many older Americans. If you're unsure about your parent's Social Security benefits or need to address any questions regarding retirement or disability benefits, contacting the Social Security Administration is a key step.

Moreover, the Department of Veterans Affairs (VA) may offer additional resources if your parent served in the military. These could include healthcare, disability compensation, and even special programs for caregivers of veterans.

Beyond these, the Older Americans Act funds a range of services designed to help older adults maintain independence. This act includes services like the National Family Caregiver Support Program, which can provide you with additional assistance.

Finally, the National Council on Aging and the Administration for Community Living are federal agencies where you can find valuable information and tools online for caregiving, health, and services for elderly citizens. Delving into these websites can provide a wealth of information, making it easier to navigate your state and federal options.

It's important to remember that you're not alone in this. Tapping into these state and federal resources can provide both you and your aging parent with the appropriate support, lighten your load, and help ensure that their later years are lived with dignity and comfort.

Online and Community Support Taking on the mantle of caregiver is a journey that, while deeply personal, need not be traversed in isolation. The beauty of the modern world lies in its interconnectedness, offering an abundance of online and community support avenues tailored to individuals engaged in the care of aging parents. In this digital era, a wealth of information and camaraderie is just a click away, and engaging with these resources can alleviate some of the weight on your shoulders.

Virtual communities and forums provide a sanctuary where one can share experiences, seek advice, and find solace in the knowledge that others understand the unique challenges faced. Websites dedicated to caregiving, such as the Family Caregiver Alliance or AARP's online community, offer discussion groups, articles, and advice specifically aimed at caregivers. The bountiful resources provided include educational webinars, interactive tools for decision-making, and directories of local services.

Legal aid, financial advice, and healthcare tips are often discussed, with professionals occasionally available to address specific concerns. These online platforms allow you to learn and grow in your role at your own pace while also providing an opportunity to contribute to the wider community by sharing your own insights and experiences.

Social media, too, can be a valuable tool for finding and building a community. Facebook groups and Twitter hashtags connect caregivers globally, facilitating a shared space for dialogue and engagement. Here, one can find motivation and encouragement through stories of triumph and perseverance, which often light the path through one's own caregiving endeavors.

Local support groups should not be overlooked, despite the ease of accessing online resources. These groups provide an opportunity to meet with others in similar situations within your community. They can be found through local hospitals, religious organizations, and community centers. Meeting face-to-face offers an invaluable level of empathy and understanding that can help you feel less alone in your caregiving journey.

Moreover, community centers and local health organizations may hold educational workshops and events that can enhance your knowledge and caregiving skills. Such events are not only informative but also provide a chance to step away from the caregiving environment, engage with the community, and recharge your emotional and mental energy.

In conclusion, there is a wide net of online and community support resources available, and they offer a diverse range of benefits. Whether it's connecting with individuals who understand your situation, accessing information pertinent to your caregiving challenges, or simply finding a space to vent and receive comfort, these resources are invaluable. While the road of caregiving is indeed demanding, remember that a world of support is at your fingertips, offering you strength and wisdom for the journey ahead.

Appendix B:
Important Documents Checklist

Taking on the role of caregiver comes with an overwhelming list of responsibilities, and one crucial aspect you'll need to manage is the organization of important documents. Having these documents in order and at your fingertips can bring a sense of control during uncertain times. It can alleviate the stress of scrambling for information when it's needed most. Here's a checklist of essential documents you'll need to gather for your aging parents:

Personal Identification and Records

- *Birth certificate:* This foundational document is essential for proving identity and is required for many legal processes.

- *Social Security card:* Needed for accessing Social Security benefits, setting up various accounts, and identity verification.

- *Passport and/or state ID:* These documents serve as primary proof of identity and citizenship.

- *Marriage certificate:* Important for spousal benefits and legal matters that pertain to marital status.

- *Military discharge information:* This is necessary for obtaining military benefits and services.

Legal Documents

- *Will:* A will conveys your parents' final wishes regarding the distribution of their estate.

- *Durable power of attorney:* It appoints someone to manage financial matters if your parents are unable to do so.

- *Advance healthcare directive:* This includes living wills and healthcare powers of attorney, guiding medical care if they become incapacitated.

- *List of authorized users:* For various accounts, ensure you have a list of who is permitted access in times of need.

Financial Records

- *Bank accounts:* Gather information on all bank accounts, including checking, savings, and safe deposit boxes.

- *Investment records:* This includes stocks, bonds, mutual funds, and retirement accounts.

- *Real estate and property deeds:* Having access to these is critical for managing or transferring real estate holdings.

- *Insurance policies:* This encompasses life, health, long-term care, home, and automobile insurance documents.

- *Credit card information:* Up-to-date records can help manage expenses and prevent fraud.

Medical Information

- *Medicare or Medicaid cards:* Essential for accessing healthcare services and coverage details.

- *Medical history:* Including past and current conditions, treatments, medications, and physician contacts.

- *Living will/advance directives:* Specifics of your parents' wishes for medical treatment in various scenarios.

- *Physician directives (DNR, POLST):* Official forms indicating wishes for life-sustaining treatments.

Miscellaneous

- *Funerary pre-planning:* If your parents have made prior arrangements, include contracts or pre-payment details.

- *Keys and passwords:* A secure list of keys, access codes, and passwords for their residences, safety deposit boxes, online accounts, and digital devices.

- *List of debts and regular bills:* Understanding their financial obligations is important for budgeting and managing expenses.

As you compile these documents, it's important to keep them in a secure yet accessible location. A fireproof safe within the home or a safety deposit box can offer protection and peace of mind. Additionally, ensure that a trusted family member, cousin, or attorney knows where to find them in case of an emergency. In the digital age, encrypted digital storage is also a safe option for keeping copies, but always prioritize security to prevent identity theft or fraud.

Organizing isn't a one-time act. Periodically revisiting and updating these documents can ensure they stay relevant and reflect the current situation, ultimately smoothening your caregiving journey.

About the Author

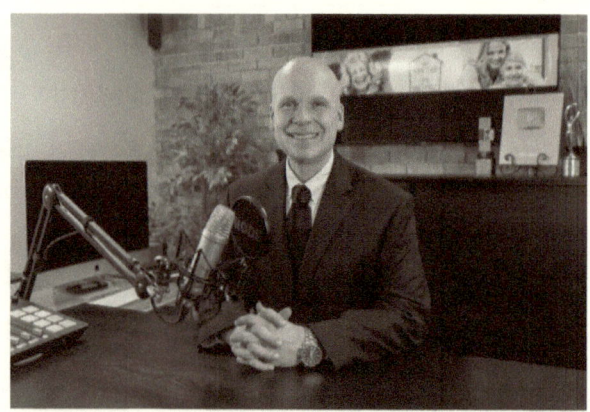

Lance A. Slatton has been described as an innovator, compassionate leader, hard working family man and passionate about what he does and where he's going. And while all of these are true, two simple words best describe Lance A. Slatton - helping others. Everything he does is about helping others and that's a pretty good way to spend your day and your life.

Slatton decided to write "The All Home Care Matters Official Family Caregivers' Guide" for exactly that reason.

"I wanted to walk a family through their caregiving journey from start to finish and help them navigate the many challenges that come with providing care for a loved one," he says. "With over 20 years of healthcare experience and through my own time as a caregiver for a loved one, I wanted to share my experiences by offering not only tips and guidelines but what they can expect on a daily basis and what's coming around the corner they might not expect. And because every case is different, we also provide numerous resources for people to use that best fit their situation as it pertains to caregiving."

Slatton has been involved in health care his entire adult life, taking EMT courses and paramedic training right after graduating from high school before beginning pursuit of a medical degree. That road eventually would hit a detour when he was needed at home to help provide care for his ailing father.

"From childhood and into my early years in adulthood, my focus has always been healthcare and finding ways to help others," Slatton says. "And while medical school didn't happen due to my experience with my father, something even more important presented itself and that was discovering how I could help others who had to provide care for their loved ones."

While helping his father, Slatton and his wife discovered they were pretty much on their own when it came to providing care. There was very little support and guidance in home care at the time and they were forced to learn on the fly and do the best they could on their own.

Armed with his "helping others" philosophy and belief there had to be a better way of providing home care, Slatton helped start Enriched Life Home Care Services (ELHCS) in 2013 in Livonia, Michigan. Since 2019, ELHCS has been named the No. 1 home care company in Michigan.

"Our name was selected so that others would know that our goal is to provide them with an 'enriched life' through our home care services," Slatton says. "Because of our compassionate and dependable care, we have been entrusted by many with their loved ones through the past nine years. We are passionate about enhancing the quality of our clients' lives!"

In May 2020, Slatton and ELHCS launched All Home Care Matters, a YouTube program and popular podcast focused on long-term care issues. The show, hosted by Slatton, has more than 122,000 YouTube subscribers and 65,000 daily podcast downloads. It was a 2023 29th annual AIVA Communicator Award Recipient (Academy of Interactive Visual Arts) and recipient of the Silver Creator Award from Google & YouTube in 2023 - given out to 0.5% of the over 80 million YouTube channels.

All Home Care Matters is focused on helping others navigate through the challenges of providing care - something Slatton didn't have during his time helping his father. As host of All Home Care Matters, Slatton is always looking for ways to help listeners and viewers to find and have the information, resources, and support that they need as they face long-term care issues and letting them know that they are not alone.

Slatton has long been passionate about providing care and resources for caregivers.

"The home care industry faces unprecedented challenges in terms of staffing and retention," he says. "To navigate these challenges successfully, home care companies need to prioritize the well-being of their caregivers. By taking the steps to do so, home care companies can attract skilled caregivers and retain them, ultimately enhancing the quality of care provided to those who depend on their services."

Slatton also serves as a member of the Board of Directors for a senior center in Monroe County, Michigan, and writes a monthly column on McKnight's Home Care News Site.

Recognizing Slatton's contributions to the industry, he was named a "50 Under 50" honoree by the New York City Journal for 2023. A testament to his visionary approach and outstanding dedication, this prestigious recognition has placed him in the ranks of some of the most influential professionals in the world.

With over 20 years of experience, Slatton, CSCM, is a seasoned professional in the healthcare industry and an award-winning visionary. His wealth of knowledge and experience, along with his innovative approach to providing care, have made him an indispensable asset in the healthcare field. And he's doing what he loves to do - helping others.

www.ingramcontent.com/pod-product-compliance
Lightning Source LLC
Chambersburg PA
CBHW030350290526
45785CB00004B/1674